301 Careers in Nursing

Joyce J. Fitzpatrick, PhD, MBA, RN, FAAN, FNAP, is Elizabeth Brooks Ford Professor of Nursing, Frances Payne Bolton School of Nursing, Case Western Reserve University (CWRU) in Cleveland, Ohio, where she was dean from 1982 through 1997. She is also adjunct professor, Department of Geriatrics, Ichan School of Medicine, Mount Sinai Hospital, New York, New York. She earned a Bachelor of Science in Nursing (Georgetown University), an MS in psychiatric–mental health nursing (The Ohio State University), a PhD in nursing (New York University), and an MBA (CWRU). In 1990, Dr. Fitzpatrick received an honorary doctorate, Doctor of Humane Letters, from Georgetown University. In 2011, she received an honorary doctorate, Doctor of Humane Letters, from Frontier University of Nursing in Hyden, Kentucky. She was elected a Fellow in the American Academy of Nursing (AAN) (1981) and a Fellow in the National Academies of Practice (1996).

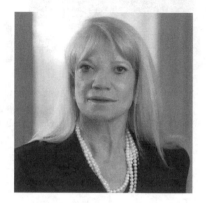

She received the *American Journal of Nursing* Book of the Year Award 20 times; the Midwest Nursing Research Society Distinguished Contribution to Nursing Research Award; The Ohio State University Distinguished Alumna Award; Sigma Theta Tau International (STTI) Elizabeth McWilliams Miller Founders Award for Excellence in Nursing Research; and New York University Division of Nursing Distinguished Alumna Award. In 1994–1995 she was the AAN/American Nurses Foundation (ANF)/ Institute of Medicine Distinguished Scholar, and in 1995 she was a Primary Care Fellow through the Bureau of Health Professions. Dr. Fitzpatrick received the ANF Distinguished Contribution to Nursing Science Award for sustained commitment and contributions to development of the discipline (2002). Recent awards include STTI Lucie Kelly Mentor Award (2003); STTI Founders Award for Leadership (2005); Fulbright Scholar at University College Cork, Cork, Ireland (2007–2008); Midwest Nursing Research Society Lifetime Achievement Award (2010); INANE Editors Award (2013); and STTI Research Hall of Fame Induction (2014). In 2016 she was named a Living Legend of the AAN.

Dr. Fitzpatrick is widely published in nursing and health care literature with over 300 publications, including more than 80 authored/edited books. She served as co-editor of the *Annual Review of Nursing Research* series, vols. 1–26, and she currently edits the journals *Applied Nursing Research, Archives of Psychiatric Nursing* and *Nursing Education Perspectives*, the official journal of the National League for Nursing. She edited three editions of the classic *Encyclopedia of Nursing Research*.

Emerson E. Ea, DNP, PhD, APRN, CNE, is clinical associate professor and director of the undergraduate program at New York University Rory Meyers College of Nursing. He obtained his Doctor of Nursing Practice degree from Case Western Reserve University and PhD from Duquesne University School of Nursing. He completed his Master of Science in Nursing from Long Island University and his Bachelor of Science in Nursing from the University of St. La Salle, Philippines. His scholarship interests include immigrant health, especially cardiovascular health among Filipino Americans, and global health and nursing education. He is an active member of the Philippine Nurses Association, the Asian American and Pacific Island Nurses Association, and the Sigma Theta Tau and Phi Kappa Phi honor societies. He was senior manager for evidence-based practice and nursing research at Mount Sinai Hospital, New York, New York, from 2011–2013; a Jonas Policy Scholar for the American Academy of Nursing Cultural Competence and Health Equity Expert Panel from 2014–2016; and he is currently a Fellow of the American Association 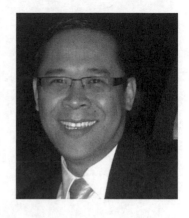 of Colleges of Nursing Leadership in Academic Nursing Program (LANP). He is board certified in nursing education by the National League for Nursing.

Dr. Ea has authored/co-authored articles on topics that relate to work- and personal-related outcomes among internationally educated nurses, Filipino immigrant health, gerontologic nursing, and nursing education and practice. He received the Nursing Research Award from the Philippine Nurses Association of New York in 2012; the New York University Rory Meyers College of Nursing Distinguished Faculty Award in 2011, the Most Outstanding Nursing Alumnus Award (Nursing Research Category) from the University of St. La Salle, Philippines; and the 2015 Asian American Pacific Islander Nurses Association Scholarship Award. He is currently board secretary for Kalusugan Coalition, an organization dedicated to creating a unified voice to improve the health of the Filipino American community in the New York/New Jersey area through network and resource development, educational activities, research, community action, and advocacy. He was recognized in 2016 by the president of the Borough of Queens, New York, for his contribution to the Filipino American community.

Laura Stark Bai, MSN, FNP-BC, RN, is the clinical nurse manager in the emergency department at Mount Sinai Medical Center in New York City. She received a Bachelor of Science in Nursing from Georgetown University in Washington, DC, and an MS from Columbia University in New York, New York. She is a board-certified family nurse practitioner and is currently enrolled in the Doctor of Nursing Practice program at the Frances Payne Bolton School of Nursing, Case Western Reserve University in Cleveland, Ohio. She was honored by the Mount Sinai emergency department residency program as Nurse of the Year in 2013 and was 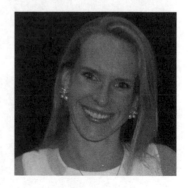 inducted into Sigma Theta Tau, the Honor Society of Nursing. She has held a number of nursing leadership positions at Mount Sinai Medical Center.

301 Careers in Nursing

JOYCE J. FITZPATRICK, PhD, MBA, RN, FAAN, FNAP

EMERSON E. EA, DNP, PhD, APRN, CNE

LAURA STARK BAI, MSN, FNP-BC, RN

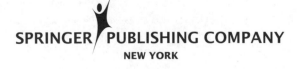

SPRINGER PUBLISHING COMPANY
NEW YORK

Springer Publishing Company, LLC
11 West 42nd Street
New York, NY 10036
www.springerpub.com

Acquisitions Editor: Joseph Morita
Composition: Exeter Premedia Services Private Ltd.

ISBN: 978-0-8261-3306-9
e-book ISBN: 978-0-8261-3308-3

17 18 19 / 5 4 3 2 1

The author and the publisher of this Work have made every effort to use sources believed to be reliable to provide information that is accurate and compatible with the standards generally accepted at the time of publication. Because medical science is continually advancing, our knowledge base continues to expand. Therefore, as new information becomes available, changes in procedures become necessary. We recommend that the reader always consult current research and specific institutional policies before performing any clinical procedure. The author and publisher shall not be liable for any special, consequential, or exemplary damages resulting, in whole or in part, from the readers' use of, or reliance on, the information contained in this book. The publisher has no responsibility for the persistence or accuracy of URLs for external or third-party Internet websites referred to in this publication and does not guarantee that any content on such websites is, or will remain, accurate or appropriate.

Library of Congress Cataloging-in-Publication Data

Names: Fitzpatrick, Joyce J., 1944- author. | Ea, Emerson E., author. | Bai,
    Laura Stark, author.
Title: 301 careers in nursing / Joyce J. Fitzpatrick, Emerson E. Ea, Laura
    Stark Bai.
Other titles: Three hundred one careers in nursing | Three hundred and one
    careers in nursing | Careers in nursing
Description: New York, NY: Springer Publishing Company, LLC, [2017] |
    Includes index.
Identifiers: LCCN 2016052490| ISBN 9780826133069 | ISBN 9780826133086 (e-book)
Subjects: | MESH: Nursing | Career Choice | Vocational Guidance | United
    States
Classification: LCC RT82 | NLM WY 16 AA1 | DDC 610.7306/9—dc23
LC record available at https://lccn.loc.gov/2016052490

Contact us to receive discount rates on bulk purchases.
We can also customize our books to meet your needs.
For more information please contact: sales@springerpub.com

Printed in the United States of America by McNaughton & Gunn.

CONTENTS

Contents

Contents

Contents

Contents

Contents

Contents

PREFACE

We, the authors of this book, are passionate about nursing and the career opportunities within the nursing profession. We have had many opportunities within our own careers to expand our roles; to contribute to quality patient care, nursing, and health care science; and to make the world a better place for patients and their families, for the communities in which we live and work, and, importantly, for the citizens of the world.

We firmly believe that there is no other career that has as much potential for personal and professional satisfaction. A career in nursing offers opportunities to care for others from infancy through older adulthood, with needs ranging from those seeking health information to those experiencing a terminal illness. Nurses work with individuals and families at their most vulnerable times of illness and have the most intimate relationships with patients. Nurses are there in time of need. They are in hospitals 24 hours a day, 7 days a week, 365 days a year, monitoring every aspect of patient care. They are in communities, delivering home care to those who are house bound due to illness or injury, providing health education in schools, in wellness centers, and in medical offices. They are aboard cruise ships and in resorts, and they transport patients, via helicopter or ambulance, when care is necessary at another facility. Nursing is all these things: listening to the cries of a newborn and the joys of the parents; being with an older woman who has fractured her hip and knows she will no longer be able to live independently; tending to the wounds of those in combat, and understanding how anxious they are to return to their loved ones at the same time they want to serve their country; soothing the pain of the person recovering from surgery; and studying the effects of new treatments for cancer, cardiovascular disease, and many other illnesses. As you will discover in this book, nurses have the choice of myriad careers. We have identified the 301 most prominent careers in nursing at this time. We have provided information so that you are introduced to opportunities within and across the careers. For example, many nurses combine careers as educators, teaching part time in schools of nursing, and expert clinicians, working clinically as advanced practice nurses in hospitals and health centers. Nurses who hold academic appointments combine the role of teacher with that of researcher. Nurses who work in management often combine their administrative work with writing and lecturing.

If you are considering a career in nursing, this book will introduce you to the wide range of career choices. You will be surprised and impressed by the many career choices available. When we talked with potential students, who over a period of time have realized that a nursing career might be right for them, they mentioned the stereotypes that are still prevalent in the public view of nursing. Indeed, strong stereotypes persist, many of which date to an earlier era when nursing required little educational preparation and much of the work was task oriented and rote, in contrast to today's complex care requiring high-level clinical judgment and skills.

If you know someone who is considering a career in nursing, this book provides an excellent overview of the potential career opportunities. Many prospective nurses are not aware of the broad range of career paths, even though they may have decided on nursing as their career choice. We often hear people say that they could never be a nurse as they do not like the "blood and guts" aspect of care. Granted, there is a dimension of the educational program that requires the nursing student to experience bloody procedures, but in many career choices there is no blood. Read about the possibilities in psychiatric or community health nursing, in historical or ethical research, or in executive positions.

If you are a guidance counselor, this book will help you learn more about the profession of nursing. You will be better prepared to advise others about the educational requirements and the competencies necessary for the specific careers.

If you are a nurse and considering a change in your career, this book will help you identify the range of opportunities and the skill sets necessary for each career. You may decide to return to school to gain more education to prepare yourself for the new career, or you may learn more about a particular career by shadowing an expert nurse who is already in that career.

HOW SHOULD YOU USE THIS BOOK TO FIND A JOB IN NURSING?

First, you should acquaint yourself with the range of possibilities: Review the table of contents for the list of career choices in nursing. Next, eliminate some of these options. If you have an interest in older adults, look first at the descriptions within geriatric nursing. If you are more interested in caring for children, a range of careers for pediatric nurses is described here. The following tips will help you in your search of a career or job within nursing:

- Consider the factors that are most important in your life. If you like being with and helping others, then a career in nursing could be right for you.
- Ask yourself why you might want to do a particular kind of work. Self-assessment is an important part of a career choice.

- Think about nursing as a career, not just a job choice. Engage in some long-range planning as well as short-term consideration of job opportunities.
- Decide if there are any parameters you wish to rule out; for example, age group.
- Consider the place of employment. Some people are petrified of hospitals, yet they might make good community health nurses.
- Select what you might consider the "top 10" careers of interest.
- Read the basic description provided for the careers that might interest you.
- Review the educational requirements for the career. If you have this educational background, you are prepared to pursue the career. If you do not have the required educational background but are still interested in the career, decide how you will become prepared. Many formal college or university programs and continuing education opportunities are available, and these often provide flexible schedules for the student or the nurse who must continue to work full time while taking classes.
- Review the core competencies needed to be successful in the career. If you do not already possess these competencies, decide how you will prepare yourself.
- Develop your résumé, highlighting the experiences and competencies that qualify you for the new career.
- Learn as much as you can about the position; access the websites that are listed for each career in order to obtain more detailed information.
- Ask others what they know about the career; plan to meet someone who is already in that career. Today the Internet makes it possible to reach out to others across the globe in order to obtain information. Schedule a time to meet with or talk with someone who is in the career of your choice. Ideally, you also would find an opportunity to "shadow" the person in his or her place of employment for at least a day.
- Networking with others is an important part of career development; you should take every opportunity to meet others and continue to network with them throughout your career development.
- Consider all opportunities carefully. Many opportunities for career advancement will come your way; consider each opportunity and decide if it fits into your overall career goals.
- Develop an action plan to get you where you want to be in your career. Make certain you have carefully considered the time frame that will be necessary for you to achieve your goals.

- Let others know—as many people as possible—that you are interested in a particular career in nursing. There is a strong network of nurses in key positions who could be helpful to you in your career search; do not hesitate to approach others for help.
- Find a mentor who can help you with your continuing professional development over the life of your career.
- Continue to build your skills in your new position and maintain your contacts for future job searches.

What binds these many nursing career opportunities are the values of the profession. Nursing is a caring profession, built on the belief that as humans we are all striving toward health. Nurses have a commitment to help individuals obtain and maintain health through education, therapeutic interventions, and evaluations of the care provided. As professionals, nurses have a societal responsibility to help others move toward health and wellness.

We believe that the descriptions of each of the careers in this book reflect the core dimensions of nursing—the caring, competence, and commitment to excellence and to serving people in their time of need. We are proud to be nurses. Through this book we want to spread the word, not only of the value of our profession, but also of the benefits to individuals who choose a career in nursing.

Joyce J. Fitzpatrick
Emerson E. Ea
Laura Stark Bai

ACCREDITATION DIRECTOR

1

BASIC DESCRIPTION
An accreditation director (or director of accreditation) is an individual who is ultimately responsible for the coordination, planning, and implementation of various initiatives to improve compliance for regulatory agencies and accreditation surveys. Accreditation directors act as the liaison between an institution and regulatory agencies leading up to, during, and after a visit to the institution. This individual manages multiple responsibilities, including but not limited to ensuring institutional compliance with regulations and initiatives; generating, analyzing, and sharing data to contribute to and support decision making; completing or reviewing reports for submission to accrediting agencies; assessing organizational policies; and more. Employment can be in health care facilities or academic institutions, and there are a number of accrediting agencies for both health care delivery and nursing education.

EDUCATIONAL REQUIREMENTS
A bachelor's degree in nursing, business, or a health care–related field is necessary. A master's degree is highly preferred for this position. Attainment of the certified professional in health care quality (CPHQ) credential is encouraged.

CORE COMPETENCIES/SKILLS NEEDED
- Strong organizational and collaborative skills
- High level of motivation
- Excellent communication skills
- Ability to lead a large group of people and delegate as needed
- Ability to understand and implement complex regulations as set by accrediting agencies
- Strong computer skills

RELATED WEBSITES AND PROFESSIONAL ORGANIZATIONS
- Accreditation Association for Ambulatory Health Care (www .aaahc.org)
- Accreditation Commission for Education in Nursing (www .acenursing.org)
- Accreditation Commission for Health Care (www.achc.org)
- American Association of Colleges of Nursing (www.aacn.nche.edu)
- Center for Improvement in Healthcare Quality (www.cihq.org)

- Community Health Accreditation Partner (www.chapinc.org)
- Healthcare Facilities Accreditation Program (www.hfap.org)
- Healthcare Quality Association on Accreditation (www.hqaa.org)
- National Association for Healthcare Quality (www.nahq.org)
- National Committee for Quality Assurance (www.ncqa.org)
- National League for Nursing (www.nln.org)
- The Joint Commission (www.jointcommission.org)
- Utilization Review Accreditation Commission (www.urac.org)

ACCREDITATION PROGRAM APPRAISER

2

BASIC DESCRIPTION

An accreditation program appraiser is a nurse–leader who reviews and assesses hospitals' applications to the American Nurses Credentialing Center (ANCC), part of the American Nurses Association (ANA) Enterprise, for Practice Transition Accreditation Program (PTAP) or Primary Accreditation. Appraisers for either program can function as either a team leader or a team member in evaluating applications.

EDUCATIONAL REQUIREMENTS

RN preparation is required and license to practice in any state, or the international equivalent to this, is necessary. A master's degree in a relevant field is needed. Prior experience with accreditation and regulatory standards is also required.

CORE COMPETENCIES/SKILLS NEEDED
- Critical thinking skills
- Thorough knowledge of accreditation and regulatory stands and up-to-date knowledge of health care policy
- Highly organized and detail oriented
- In-depth understanding of standards of practice for nursing
- Strong interpersonal skills
- Excellent written and oral communication skills
- Active listening skills
- Good computer skills
- Ability to work collaboratively and independently
- Understanding of adult education
- Strong judgment skills
- Ability to analyze and synthesize information effectively and efficiently

RELATED WEBSITES AND PROFESSIONAL ORGANIZATIONS
- American Nurses Association (www.nursingworld.org)
- American Nurses Credentialing Center (www.nursecredentialing.org)

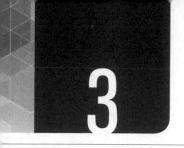

3 ACCREDITATION SPECIALIST

BASIC DESCRIPTION

An accreditation specialist works as part of a team at health care facilities or as part of a university to ensure organizational compliance with quality standards and regulations as set by various regulatory agencies. Accreditation specialists can work with management or frontline staff to implement or monitor initiatives that improve practices or ensure adherence to institutional policies that meet regulatory standards. They may also collect, analyze, and share data that can be used to improve this process.

EDUCATIONAL REQUIREMENTS

A bachelor's degree in nursing, business, or a health care–related field is necessary. A master's degree is highly preferred for this position. Attainment of the certified professional in health care quality (CPHQ) credential is available and encouraged for those seeking to work with health care organizations.

CORE COMPETENCIES/SKILLS NEEDED

- Educational skills
- Strong organizational and collaborative skills
- High level of motivation
- Excellent communication skills
- Ability to understand and implement complex regulations as set by accrediting agencies
- Strong computer skills

RELATED WEBSITES AND PROFESSIONAL ORGANIZATIONS

- Accreditation Association for Ambulatory Health Care, Inc. (www.aaahc.org)
- Accreditation Commission for Health Care (www.achc.org)
- American Association of Colleges of Nursing (www.aacn.nche.edu)
- Center for Improvement in Healthcare Quality (www.cihq.org)
- Community Health Accreditation Program (www.chapinc.org)
- Healthcare Facilities Accreditation Partner (www.hfap.org)
- Healthcare Quality Association on Accreditation (www.hqaa.org)
- National Association for Healthcare Quality (www.nahq.org)
- National Committee for Quality Assurance (www.ncqa.org)
- National League for Nursing (www.nln.org)
- The Joint Commission (www.jointcommission.org)
- Utilization Review Accreditation Commission (www.urac.org)

ACTIVIST

BASIC DESCRIPTION

An activist advocates for a specific cause and is involved in political movements to promote change. It is important that nurses function as activists in campaigning for improvements for the profession and for patients, families, and communities. Some examples of causes that nurses support are safe staffing, health care reform, patient safety, and workplace safety. The level of involvement can vary from simply writing letters to Congress to participating in protests to volunteering on campaigns.

EDUCATIONAL REQUIREMENTS

There is no educational requirement to be involved in activism. To be an activist for nursing, one should be an RN with a minimum of a bachelor's degree in nursing.

CORE COMPETENCIES/SKILLS NEEDED

- Ability to professionally voice an opinion
- Excellent communication skills
- Persistence, courage, and patience
- Creativity
- Critical thinking skills
- Passion about the cause
- Knowledge of state and federal laws that affect health care
- Knowledge of political and legislative processes and procedures
- Knowledge of the U.S. health care system

RELATED WEBSITES AND PROFESSIONAL ORGANIZATIONS

- American Nurses Association RN Action (www.rnaction.org)
- Specialty nursing organizations
- State nurses associations

5 ACUPUNCTURIST NURSE

BASIC DESCRIPTION
An acupuncturist nurse is a holistic practitioner based on traditional Chinese medicine's concept of integrative health. The acupuncturist nurse uses needles, heat, or pressure to promote wellness, health, and balance. Acupuncturist nurses are employed by ambulatory centers and holistic care centers.

EDUCATIONAL REQUIREMENTS
RN preparation is preferred; certification is available from the National Certification Commission for Acupuncture and Oriental Medicine.

CORE COMPETENCIES/SKILLS NEEDED
Additional education and training in holistic medicine are required.

- Knowledge of anatomy and Centers for Disease Control and Prevention infection control standards
- Excellent communication and interpersonal skills

RELATED WEBSITES AND PROFESSIONAL ORGANIZATIONS
- American Association of Acupuncture and Oriental Medicine (www.aaaomonline.org)
- National Certification Commission for Acupuncture and Oriental Medicine (www.nccaom.org)

ACUTE CARE NURSE PRACTITIONER

6

BASIC DESCRIPTION

Acute care nurse practitioners are advanced practice nurses who specialize in providing care for acutely ill patients in a variety of settings. The environment in which acute care nurse practitioners function is very intense and dramatic. Some of the characteristics of an acute care nurse practitioner's work include coordinating patient care, assessing the patient's health history, ordering diagnostic tests, performing therapeutic procedures, and prescribing medications. Possibilities for work exist in these settings:

- Emergency rooms
- Operating rooms
- Critical care units
- Transplant units

EDUCATIONAL REQUIREMENTS

Master of Science in Nursing (MSN) with advanced practice certification as an acute care nurse practitioner is required. Graduate programs are generally 2 years long. The number of schools that offer this specialty is limited; therefore, entry into these programs is competitive. Certification is available from the American Nurses Credentialing Center or the American Association of Critical-Care Nurses.

CORE COMPETENCIES/SKILLS NEEDED

- Technical competency involving use of complex and computerized equipment
- Knowledge of regulating ventilators
- Knowledge of hemodynamic monitoring
- Skill to obtain blood samples from central lines
- Interpersonal competency dealing with patients and their families in life-threatening situations
- Ability to work with interdisciplinary teams
- Extensive experience and expertise in assessing and managing acutely ill patients

RELATED WEBSITES AND PROFESSIONAL ORGANIZATIONS

- American Association of Critical-Care Nurses (www.aacn.org)
- American Association of Nurse Practitioners (www.aanp.org)
- American Nurses Credentialing Center (www.nursecredentialing.org)
- Nurse Practitioner Associates for Continuing Education (www.npace.org)
- Nurse Practitioner Support Services (www.nurse.net)

ADDICTIONS COUNSELOR

BASIC DESCRIPTION
Nurses who are addictions counselors work in organizations that specialize in helping clients overcome addictive disorders. Treatment programs exist in all regions of the country. Chemical dependency is a major health problem, and nurses work with clients to help them learn more effective ways of coping.

EDUCATIONAL REQUIREMENTS
Bachelor of Science in Nursing is preferred with certification as a certified addictions registered nurse (CARN). Three years' experience as an RN is necessary for CARN certification. Within the 5 years prior to the application for certification, a minimum of 4,000 hours (2 years) of nursing experience related to addictions is required. There is also an advanced practice certification that requires the Master of Science in Nursing degree.

CORE COMPETENCIES/SKILLS NEEDED
- Excellent interpersonal and counseling skills
- Good interviewing techniques
- Strong assessment skills
- Counseling ability
- Compassion and empathy
- Interest in mental health
- Ability to work in interdisciplinary teams

RELATED WEBSITES AND PROFESSIONAL ORGANIZATIONS
- American Nurses Association Peer Assistance Program (www.ana.org)
- International Nurses Society on Addictions (www.intnsa.org)

ADMINISTRATOR/MANAGER

BASIC DESCRIPTION

Nurse administrators and executive directors are needed in numerous organizations. Knowledge of finance, law, human resources, and related topics improve the systems necessary for the advancement of health care administration and delivery. Nurses are managers, administrators, and executive directors in hospitals, nursing homes, colleges and universities, and health maintenance organizations. Administrators employ, direct, evaluate, promote, and terminate employees. An administrator must have the ability to analyze budgets and make certain that financial plans are consistent with the organizational mission and goals. Work hours are often long, but the rewards are gratifying in shaping the future of the organization, the delivery of care, and the profession.

EDUCATIONAL REQUIREMENTS

Bachelor of Science in Nursing is now the entry-level degree. The majority of high-level nursing executives hold a Master of Science in Nursing or an MBA. In addition, many nurse executives are certified in administration through the American Nurses Credentialing Center.

CORE COMPETENCIES/SKILLS NEEDED
- Human resource knowledge
- Excellent interpersonal skills
- Ability to communicate clearly and persuasively
- Leadership skills
- Self-confidence
- Budgeting and finance skills
- Writing skills
- Strong work ethic
- Managerial competencies

RELATED WEBSITES AND PROFESSIONAL ORGANIZATIONS
- American College of Healthcare Executives (www.ache.org)
- American Nurses Association (www.ana.org)
- American Nurses Credentialing Center (www.nursecredentialing.org)
- American Organization of Nurse Executives (www.aone.org)

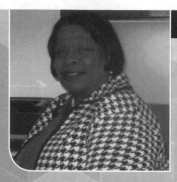

 PROFILE: LORNA GREEN
Clinical Nurse Manager,
Geropsychiatry Unit

1. What is your educational background in nursing (and other areas) and what formal credentials do you hold?

I am a clinical nurse manager at a major medical center where I have been employed for the past 35 years. My experience includes 9 years as a general duty psychiatric nurse, working with geriatric, adult, and adolescent patients with various psychiatric diagnoses and symptoms/behaviors, 2 years as senior clinical nurse, and 24 years as a clinical nurse manager. My credentials include an associate degree in nursing; a BSN, cum laude; and an MSN.

2. How did you first become interested in your current career?

As far back as I can remember, I wanted to be a nurse. During my early childhood, I saw my mother, aunts, and neighborhood women minister to friends and relatives who became ill. They provided whatever care was needed for as long as it was needed, without payment or other expectations. All care was rendered at home. Only one doctor was available to provide care for all the people on our island, and the nearest hospital was accessible only by boat or by small plane in the later years. Without the diagnosis, care, and support of neighbors, friends, and relatives, many people would have suffered and died. Therefore, I do not think that I ever "became interested" in nursing; I believe that I was born into it. How fortunate for me that my family, culture, and circumstances of birth allowed me to recognize and develop my passion at a young age. It would not be an exaggeration to state that nursing is not only my profession, it is truly my vocation and one of the most important reasons I am on this Earth.

3. What are the most rewarding aspects of your career?

Every day in nursing is rewarding in some way for me. Specifically, though, one of the most rewarding days in my life is the day I assumed responsibility

Continued

of the geropsychiatry unit. The unit presented myriad challenges. Among the most difficult was its reputation for not being consumer oriented and the lack of cohesion among staff. Interpersonal relationships were fraught with conflict at times. I am proud to say that through hard work and compromise, we have turned the unit around. We now frequently receive complimentary letters from patients and their families. Doctors, nurses, and other staff members have voiced their appreciation for the improved environment. I take great pride and personal fulfillment in my contributions and continually work hard to seek further enhancements to achieve total consumer and staff satisfaction.

4. What advice would you give to others contemplating a career such as yours?

The most important advice I would impart to a nurse considering a career in administration or management would be to spend time at the bedside, involved in direct patient care as a staff nurse to broaden your knowledge base and gain perspective. Do not jump into the leadership role prematurely. As you experience and develop more fully, more resources will become available to you. When you take on additional responsibilities in a leadership role, this will boost your confidence level and the confidence of others in you when you are making critical decisions.

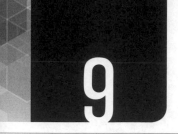

9 ADULT DAY CARE DIRECTOR

BASIC DESCRIPTION
An adult day care director coordinates, manages, and evaluates care and services to residents of an adult day care program. Residents of adult day care programs are adults who need some assistance in performing activities of daily living such as grooming and other personal care needs. As director of the program, the nurse also monitors the institution's compliance to regulatory standards and is responsible for the oversight of the institution's budget, hiring, and other personnel-related functions.

EDUCATIONAL REQUIREMENTS
RN preparation and a Bachelor of Science in Nursing are required; master's degree preparation is highly preferred and at least 3 to 5 years of experience in geriatric nursing is also preferred.

CORE COMPETENCIES/SKILLS NEEDED
- Excellent leadership and management skills
- Knowledge of federal and state regulatory standards that pertain to adult day care management
- Excellent interpersonal and communication skills
- Knowledge of budgeting and fiscal management

RELATED WEBSITE AND PROFESSIONAL ORGANIZATION
- National Adult Day Services Association (www.nadsa.org)

ADULT–GERONTOLOGY CLINICAL NURSE SPECIALIST

BASIC DESCRIPTION
The adult–gerontology clinical nurse specialist is an advanced practice nurse who is an expert in diagnosing, managing, and treating adult–gerontology patients. Adult–gerontology nurses provide direct patient care while acting as a special resource for frontline clinical nurses. They are experts in geriatric care and are able to provide guidance and consultation to the staff in complex clinical situations that are unique to the adult–geriatric population. They also play a role in patient and family education. Employment can be found in multiple venues, including hospitals, nursing homes, skilled nursing facilities, outpatient clinics or practices. Adult–gerontology clinical nurse specialists can work in research, administration, education, or clinical practice.

EDUCATIONAL REQUIREMENTS
RN preparation and a bachelor's degree in nursing are required. A master's degree as an adult–gerontology clinical nurse specialist is also required. Certification is available through the American Nurses Credentialing Center.

CORE COMPETENCIES/SKILLS NEEDED
- Basic computer skills
- High energy level and superior interpersonal skills
- Understanding of organizational structure
- Technical competencies involving use of complex equipment
- Excellent and effective communication
- Educational and teaching skills
- High level of clinical competency
- Self-confidence and strong leadership skills
- Thorough knowledge of diagnosis and treatment of psychiatric health problems
- Excellent coordination skills

RELATED WEBSITES AND PROFESSIONAL ORGANIZATIONS
- American Board of Nursing Specialties (www.nursingcertification.org)
- American Nurses Credentialing Center (www.nursecredentialing.org)
- National Association of Clinical Nurse Specialists (www.nacns.org)

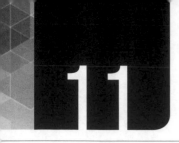

ADULT–GERONTOLOGY PRIMARY CARE NURSE PRACTITIONER

BASIC DESCRIPTION
Adult–gerontology primary care nurse practitioners are advanced practice nurses who promote wellness and prevent diseases among adults of all ages. They are primary care providers who conduct wellness checkups and manage acute and chronic health conditions. Work environments include private practice, community health centers, health clinics, assisted living facilities, rehabilitation centers, and more.

EDUCATIONAL REQUIREMENTS
RN preparation and a Master of Science in Nursing with advanced practice certification as an adult–gerontology primary care nurse practitioner are required. Certification is available through the American Association of Nurse Practitioners and American Nurses Credentialing Center. Basic life support and advanced cardiac life support certifications are also necessary.

CORE COMPETENCIES/SKILLS NEEDED
- Diagnosis and management of patients' health and illness status
- Ability to interpret diagnostic tests
- Ability to establish and maintain rapport with patients
- Ability to make referrals as needed for specialized care
- Coordination of patient care through the health care system

RELATED WEBSITES AND PROFESSIONAL ORGANIZATIONS
- American Association of Nurse Practitioners (www.aanp.org)
- American Nurses Credentialing Center (www.nursecredentialing.org)
- Gerontological Advanced Practice Nurses Association (www.gapna.org)
- National Gerontological Nursing Association (www.ngna.org)

ADULT NURSE PRACTITIONER

BASIC DESCRIPTION

Adult nurse practitioners are advanced practice nurses who specialize in providing primary care to adults in a variety of settings, such as hospitals, outpatient clinics, ambulatory care settings, physicians' offices, community-based clinics, and health care agencies. The adult nurse practitioner functions as a primary care provider and focuses on maintaining health and wellness in acute and chronic illnesses. Some of the characteristics of the work are:

- Teaching patients to manage chronic conditions
- Assessing the patient's health history and status
- Ordering diagnostic tests
- Performing therapeutic procedures
- Prescribing medications

EDUCATIONAL REQUIREMENTS

A Master of Science in Nursing is required with advanced practice certification as an adult nurse practitioner. Certification as adult health clinical nurse specialist (CNS), another advanced practice role, is available from the American Nurses Credentialing Center. Graduate programs are generally 2 years long.

CORE COMPETENCIES/SKILLS NEEDED
- Health assessment skills
- Interpersonal skills
- Ability to work in interdisciplinary teams
- Knowledge of acute and chronic diseases
- Health promotion knowledge and skills
- Knowledge of primary care provider role
- Extensive experience and expertise in assessing and managing patients in primary care settings

RELATED WEBSITES AND PROFESSIONAL ORGANIZATIONS
- American Association of Nurse Practitioners (www.aanp.org)
- American Nurses Credentialing Center (www.nursecredentialing.org)
- Nurse Practitioner Associates for Continuing Education (www.npace.org)
- Nurse Practitioner Support Services (www.npcentral.net)

13 ADULT PSYCHIATRIC– MENTAL HEALTH CLINICAL NURSE SPECIALIST

BASIC DESCRIPTION

Adult psychiatric–mental health clinical nurse specialists are advanced practice nurses who are expert in diagnosing, managing, and treating adult psychiatric patients. They provide direct patient care while acting as a special resource for frontline clinical nurses. Responsibilities include providing guidance to clinical nurses in psychiatric units, consulting on treatment plans, collaborating with psychiatrists, and maintaining a high quality of care. They are heavily involved in providing patient and family education, participating in crisis intervention, and coordinating care and follow-up for patients. Employment can be found in inpatient psychiatric–mental health units, outpatient psychiatric clinics, and behavioral health centers.

EDUCATIONAL REQUIREMENTS

RN preparation is required as is a master's degree as an adult psychiatric–mental health clinical nurse specialist. Certification is available through the American Nurses Credentialing Center.

CORE COMPETENCIES/SKILLS NEEDED

- Basic computer skills
- High energy level
- Superior interpersonal skills
- Excellent and effective verbal communication
- Ability to connect effectively with patients, families, and frontline staff
- Educational skills
- Good leadership skills
- Thorough knowledge of diagnosis and treatment of psychiatric health problems
- Excellent coordination of health care team members

RELATED WEBSITES AND PROFESSIONAL ORGANIZATIONS

- American Nurses Credentialing Center (www.nursecredentialing.org)
- National Association of Clinical Nurse Specialists (www.nacns.org)

ADULT PSYCHIATRIC–MENTAL HEALTH NURSE PRACTITIONER

BASIC DESCRIPTION
Dealing with adult patients, adult psychiatric–mental health nurse practitioners assess, diagnose, and manage mental health issues that include bipolar disorders, schizophrenia, depression, and anxiety. They may have additional training in psychotherapy or any other behavioral treatment modalities.

EDUCATIONAL REQUIREMENTS
RN preparation and nurse practitioner certification are required. Certification from the American Nurses Credentialing Center also is available as a clinical nurse specialist, another advanced practice nursing specialty role in psychiatric and mental health. Experience as a mental health RN is preferred.

CORE COMPETENCIES/SKILLS NEEDED
- Advanced knowledge in mental health
- Sensitivity to patients and their families
- Excellent verbal and written communication skills
- Knowledge in psychopharmacology and behavioral science therapy

RELATED WEBSITES AND PROFESSIONAL ORGANIZATIONS
- American Nurses Credentialing Center (www.nursingcredentialing.org)
- American Psychiatric Nurses Association (www.apna.org)
- International Society of Psychiatric–Mental Health Nurses (www.ispn-psych.org)

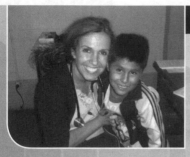

 PROFILE: MARIANNE TARRAZA

Adult Psychiatric–Mental Health Nurse Practitioner

1. What is your educational background in nursing (and other areas) and what formal credentials do you hold?

My original nursing education was at a hospital-based diploma program in the Boston area. After receiving my diploma and becoming an RN, I spent several years obtaining my Bachelor of Science in Nursing (BSN). At the time there were no programs designed for an RN-to-BSN transition, so I had to take many of my original nursing courses for a second time. I ultimately obtained a BSN and quickly moved on to a master's degree in nursing with a specialization in psychiatric nursing. I am currently certified as an adult psychiatric nurse practitioner.

2. How did you first become interested in your current career?

I began my nursing career in medical–surgical nursing and psychiatry. I worked primarily as a staff nurse on a large surgical unit and per diem on the psychiatric unit. I then moved on to various surgical disciplines, including vascular surgery, intensive care, and noninvasive vascular technology. Since there was a research component to these positions, when I later moved to Maine I worked as the research coordinator in the OB/GYN department. This position was not necessarily what I had chosen but I had young children and this work allowed me the flexibility to care for my children. While participating in clinical research, the nurse in me connected to the lived experiences of the patients so much so that when I decided to return for graduate work, I returned to my psychiatric roots and concentrated on mental health. I was primarily interested in medical illnesses that were comorbid with psychiatric disorders. I planned on a practice that was focused primarily on psychotherapy; however, during my training I became increasingly fascinated with psychopharmacology, which now is a significant component in my clinical work.

Continued

3. What are the most rewarding aspects of your career?

There are so many rewarding aspects of my career path—it is difficult to say which have been the most rewarding. Even the difficulties within my journey have been rewarding to me since they have led to other aspects that have turned out to be exceptional.

Mental health crosses all disciplines. Whether it is purely a psychiatric disorder, medical comorbidity, or a social/behavioral perspective, there is a mental health component. This is the most rewarding aspect of my career. I have the opportunity to examine relationships, coping behavior, and health from the sphere of the self.

This has also led me to participate in volunteer medical missionary work. I spend time annually working in impoverished areas in South America. The opportunity and, more importantly, the privilege of spending time in these areas have impacted me in a life-changing way. Specifically, how I approach patient care, administrative duties, nursing opportunities, and my own sense of self have been touched and realigned in an irreplaceable way.

4. What advice would you give to someone contemplating the same career path in nursing?

"Nursing has been good to me" is my favorite personal quote. Nursing has provided me with the opportunity throughout my life to attend to my personal needs while fulfilling my professional promise. I began as a naïve teenager who wanted to "help people" and continue with that mission in mind whenever I take on a new opportunity. It is to that end that I know that I have made an impact on the lives of others, even if only for a moment.

There are many avenues in which to consider how to enter nursing, all with strengths and weaknesses. To enter nursing with the knowledge that there is nothing impossible in this profession, the difference one can make in the lives of others, is an endowed privilege. I would suggest having a personal vision that is composed of possibilities now, in the near future, and in the distant future so that nothing that one does at any point is no less than breathtaking!

ALLERGY–IMMUNOLOGY NURSE

BASIC DESCRIPTION
Allergy–immunology nurses focus on the care of patients with chronic allergic conditions. These conditions include asthma, allergic rhinitis, urticaria, and atopic dermatitis. Duties include providing direct patient care and health education and, in most cases, administrative responsibilities such as those of an allergy office manager.

EDUCATIONAL REQUIREMENTS
RN preparation and basic life support certification are required. An allergy RN can obtain certification in asthma education by the National Asthma Educator Certification Board.

CORE COMPETENCIES/SKILLS NEEDED
- Strong assessment and interpersonal skills
- Ability to work with other members of the health care team
- Excellent organizational skills
- Advanced knowledge in allergy treatment and management, such as allergy desensitization therapy

RELATED WEBSITES AND PROFESSIONAL ORGANIZATIONS
- American Academy of Allergy Asthma and Immunology (www.aaaai.org)
- Association of Asthma Educators (www.asthmaeducators.org)
- National Asthma Educator Certification Board (www.naecb.org)

AMBULATORY CARE NURSE

16

BASIC DESCRIPTION

An ambulatory care nurse works as part of a multidisciplinary health care team to provide primary care to a specific population. Depending on the role the nurse plays within the ambulatory center, the work activities will differ. A triage nurse may work primarily in a walk-in area or over the telephone assessing the patients and determining the priority with which they must be seen or referred. Working with a multidisciplinary team entails gathering a medical history and information about the chief complaint and checking vital signs. Once the practitioner has seen the patient, the nurse will perform follow-up treatment, such as drawing labs, teaching the patient regarding the condition, and discharge instructions.

EDUCATIONAL REQUIREMENTS

RN preparation is required; certification is available from the American Nurses Credentialing Center.

CORE COMPETENCIES/SKILLS NEEDED

- Knowledge of illnesses and symptoms including diagnosis and management
- Experience with triage
- Strong assessment and organizational skills
- Communication skills
- Ability to collaborate and function as a member of a multidisciplinary team
- Ability to function in a fast-paced environment
- Interest in working with a diverse population

RELATED WEBSITES AND PROFESSIONAL ORGANIZATIONS

- American Academy of Ambulatory Care Nursing (www.aaacn.org)
- American Nurses Credentialing Center (www.nursecredenting.org)

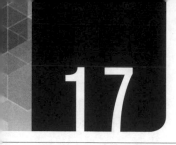

ANTICOAGULATION NURSE

BASIC DESCRIPTION

An anticoagulation nurse is responsible for monitoring patients in ambulatory care settings who are on anticoagulant therapy, such as Coumadin, based on clinical standards and protocols. Other responsibilities include anticoagulant medication administration, point-of-care testing, and health education to patients and families regarding instructions for medication and care related to anticoagulation therapy.

EDUCATIONAL REQUIREMENTS

RN preparation and several years of experience in acute or ambulatory care are required. Basic life support certification and completion of an anticoagulation management certification course are highly desirable. Certification is provided by the National Certification Board for Anticoagulation Providers.

CORE COMPETENCIES/SKILLS NEEDED

- Excellent communication skills
- Strong computer skills
- Knowledge of the complex interactions among food, supplements, electrolytes, and drugs with anticoagulant therapy
- Knowledge of physiology of hemostasis and its related pathophysiology

RELATED WEBSITE AND PROFESSIONAL ORGANIZATION

- National Certification Board for Anticoagulation Providers (www.ncbap.org)

AROMATHERAPIST NURSE

18

BASIC DESCRIPTION
An aromatherapist nurse is a specially trained nurse who uses the soothing and healing properties of scents from essential oils to relieve pain and other discomforts, decrease stress, elevate moods, relax, and treat conditions. Their services are employed in many health care settings such as health spas, holistic health centers, and hospitals.

EDUCATIONAL REQUIREMENTS
An RN certification is preferred; basic life support certification is required.

CORE COMPETENCIES/SKILLS NEEDED
- Knowledge of essential oils and their effects
- Knowledge of Centers for Disease Control and Prevention infection control principles and standards
- Excellent communication and interpersonal skills

RELATED WEBSITES AND PROFESSIONAL ORGANIZATIONS
- American Holistic Nurses Association (www.ahna.org)
- National Association of Holistic Aromatherapy (www.naha.org)
- National Center for Complementary and Integrative Health (nccih.nih.gov)

19   ATTORNEY

BASIC DESCRIPTION
Nurse attorneys engage in a range of legal activities including the following:

- Provide legal consult; prosecute/defend cases; may represent individuals, patients, health professionals, or institutions
- Provide depositions and court testimony
- Engage in legal research
- Define standards of care
- Serve as quality-of-care experts for hospitals and other health care institutions
- Review cases
- Define applicable standards of care
- Organize records
- Research the literature
- Provide behind-the-scenes or up-front consultations
- Interview clients and witnesses
- Prepare exhibits
- Prepare questions for depositions and court

EDUCATIONAL REQUIREMENTS
RN preparation and juris doctor (JD) degree are required.

CORE COMPETENCIES/SKILLS NEEDED
- Logical thinking skills
- Knowledge of judicial system and health care legislation

RELATED WEBSITES AND PROFESSIONAL ORGANIZATIONS
- American Association of Nurse Attorneys (www.taana.org)
- Registered Nurse Experts, Inc. (www.rnexperts.com)

PROFILE: CAROL ANN ROE
Nurse Attorney and City Council Member

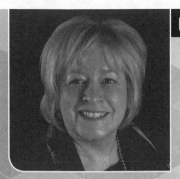

1. What is your educational background in nursing (and other areas) and what formal credentials do you hold?

I received my diploma and worked on my bachelor's degree in nursing soon afterward. After some more years in practice, I received a master's degree in nursing, majoring in medical–surgical nursing with a minor in nursing administration. In recognition of the increased interface between health care and law, I obtained a JD. I am admitted to the practice of law in Ohio and the U.S. Supreme Court. Additionally, I have a Certificate of Authority from the Ohio Board of Nursing as a clinical nurse specialist (CNS).

2. How did you first become interested in your current career?

I have been politically active as a citizen and nurse my entire adult life. My parents instilled in me the values of caring for others and participating as a citizen in the community. Those values led to my lobbying elected officials and working on campaigns. Over the years I became known in political circles as the "go-to" person for health care–related issues. I also mentored other nurses in the political process and worked to identify nurses who would run for office. I was approached in 2014 by politically active women I know to seek a seat on the Cuyahoga County Council. I did not win the seat but ran for Cleveland Heights City Council in 2015 and won.

I chose to go to law school to enhance my skills as an advocate for both the profession and the patients we serve. My preparation in law has equipped me with the knowledge and skills to provide continuing education to nurses about legal issues in practice. It has also deepened my understanding of the need to critically examine all sides of an issue. My full-time job as a risk manager and compliance officer is a blend of both nursing and law.

Continued

PROFILE: CAROL ANN ROE
Continued

3. What are the most rewarding aspects of your career?

I am fortunate to have so many rewarding aspects in my career. I have had a variety of jobs (staff nurse, nursing administrator, CNS in long-term care, lobbyist, nursing regulator, faculty member, risk manager/compliance officer) and have been constantly stimulated to learn. Another rewarding aspect has been to see some nurses become more involved in direct political activity as a result of my mentoring efforts. I am also proud of those nurses who have continued their education as a result of my influence.

I have had the privilege of meeting and talking with two U.S. presidents more than once in my political involvement. As the lobbyist for the Ohio Nurses Association, I was one of the leaders in the efforts to expand the role of advanced practice registered nurses. It is a gratifying experience to impact the system in a way that enhances the delivery of health care services.

4. What advice would you give to someone contemplating the same career path in nursing?

If a person wants to pursue a political career, I would remind him or her that politics is about the allocation of scarce resources and it exists all around us, not just in government. It is also essential to recognize that compromise is an essential component of the process. If one is not willing to think about what one can give up, the process can be frustrating and unrewarding. I also found that campaigning as a nurse was an asset. I stressed that my preparation as a nurse taught me to listen to what was not being said as well as what was stated.

In pursuing a law career, one needs to recognize that law school curricula are not necessarily based on a conceptual framework, as in nursing school. I found it challenging to find a link between property law and criminal law.

AUTHOR/WRITER 20

BASIC DESCRIPTION

An author or writer is an RN who works in any area of writing. This written material may be used in research, biomedical research, education, training, sales and marketing, and other medical mediums and communication forms. Writers need the ability at times to work with voluminous technical information. Authors or editors may write for medical and general interest publications, freelance, professional organizations, and medical trade journals.

EDUCATIONAL REQUIREMENTS

RN preparation is required; a Bachelor of Science in Nursing, or higher, is often also required.

CORE COMPETENCIES/SKILLS NEEDED

- Good command of the English language
- Ability to work alone
- Ability to meet deadlines
- Excellent writing skills
- Health care–related knowledge

RELATED WEBSITES AND PROFESSIONAL ORGANIZATIONS

- American Medical Writers Association (www.amwa.org)
- Registered Nurse Experts, Inc. (www.rnexperts.com)

21 BARIATRIC NURSE

BASIC DESCRIPTION
A bariatric nurse provides holistic care to patients who have a diagnosis of morbid obesity. It also includes care of patients undergoing bariatric surgeries.

EDUCATIONAL REQUIREMENTS
RN preparation and basic life support certification are required; certification as a bariatric nurse is offered by the American Society for Metabolic and Bariatric Surgery.

CORE COMPETENCIES/SKILLS NEEDED
- Excellent assessment and critical thinking skills
- Sensitivity to the needs of patients who are morbidly obese, and their families
- Knowledge of evidence-based practice related to bariatric medicine

RELATED WEBSITES AND PROFESSIONAL ORGANIZATIONS
- American Society for Metabolic and Bariatric Surgery (www.asbs.org)
- Obesity Society (obesity.org/home)

BARIATRIC NURSE PRACTITIONER

BASIC DESCRIPTION
A bariatric nurse practitioner (NP) provides either inpatient or outpatient care to patients who are morbidly obese. Aside from providing direct care, a bariatric nurse practitioner provides patient teaching, evaluates patient progress after bariatric surgery and alters plan if needed, and prepares patients for discharge in collaboration with the bariatric surgery team.

EDUCATIONAL REQUIREMENTS
RN preparation and NP certification, basic life support certification, and a Master of Science in Nursing (MSN) are required. Advanced training and certification as a bariatric nurse are available by the American Society for Metabolic and Bariatric Surgery and by the American Board of Bariatric Medicine.

CORE COMPETENCIES/SKILLS NEEDED
- Previous experience in bariatric surgery, general surgery, or internal medicine
- Excellent assessment and critical thinking skills
- Sensitivity to the needs of patients who are morbidly obese, and their families
- Knowledge of evidence-based practice related to bariatric medicine

RELATED WEBSITES AND PROFESSIONAL ORGANIZATIONS
- American Board of Bariatric Medicine; American Board of Obesity Medicine (www.abom.org)
- American Society for Metabolic and Bariatric Surgery (www.asbs.org)
- Obesity Medicine Association (https://asmbs.org)

23 BED MANAGEMENT COORDINATOR

BASIC DESCRIPTION
A bed coordinator is a nurse with clinical experience who works to facilitate hospital throughput by assigning patients to their hospital beds. They assess patients' needs and develop an appropriate plan to prioritize bed placement that meets the patients' specialty needs (i.e., intensive care, telemetry monitoring, isolation). They also work directly with clinical nurses to help expedite patient movement to ensure efficiency and optimal coordination.

EDUCATIONAL REQUIREMENTS
A bachelor's degree in nursing or a health-related field is required. Clinical experience in an acute care setting is preferred.

CORE COMPETENCIES/SKILLS NEEDED
- Understanding of different levels of acuity and levels of medical care
- Knowledge of patient flow through the hospital in various situations
- Ability to think critically and prioritize
- Knowledge of hospital operations
- Creativity
- Team orientedness
- Excellent communication skills
- Excellent computer skills

RELATED WEBSITES AND PROFESSIONAL ORGANIZATIONS
There are no related websites or organizations.

BIOFEEDBACK NURSE

24

BASIC DESCRIPTION
Biofeedback nurses assist patients to promote and improve health and manage symptoms by using signals from the body. Biofeedback, as a primary treatment modality or as adjunct therapy, is used to manage chronic pain, stress, anxiety, urinary incontinence, asthma, and headache.

EDUCATIONAL REQUIREMENTS
RN preparation is required; certification is offered by the Biofeedback Certification International Alliance.

CORE COMPETENCIES/SKILLS NEEDED
- Knowledge of operation of equipment used in biofeedback therapy
- Knowledge of the physiologic manifestations of stress, pain, and other chronic conditions
- Excellent interpersonal and communication skills
- Good computer skills and knowledge of electronic health record documentation

RELATED WEBSITES AND PROFESSIONAL ORGANIZATIONS
- Association for Applied Psychophysiology and Biofeedback, Inc. (www.aapb.org)
- Biofeedback Certification International Alliance (www.bcia.org)

25

BOARD MEMBER

BASIC DESCRIPTION

The board of directors of an organization consists of a group of elected or appointed people who together envision and oversee the strategic mission and goals of an organization or company. The board's responsibilities generally include oversight of finances and budgeting, performance of the organization and its executive leaders, assurance of continued improvement of quality and services, and organizational governance for policies and objectives.

EDUCATION REQUIREMENTS

A bachelor's and/or master's degree in health care or business is preferred to serve on a board of directors.

CORE COMPETENCIES/SKILLS NEEDED

- Highly organized and focused
- Excellent leadership and management skills
- Professionalism
- Creativity and ability to problem solve
- Ability to be objective and assertive
- Strong communication and interpersonal skills
- Thorough understanding of budgeting and financial management
- Ability to collaborate and work well with a team
- Deep understanding of the organization's culture, policies, mission, and goals

RELATED WEBSITES AND PROFESSIONAL ORGANIZATIONS

- American Organization of Nurse Executives (www.aone.org)
- Sigma Theta Tau International (www.nursingsociety.org)

BONE MARROW TRANSPLANT NURSE

26

BASIC DESCRIPTION

Bone marrow transplant (BMT) nurses manage patients receiving this special therapy to treat cancer, anemia, or other diseases that affect the bone marrow. In addition to basic nursing care, these nurses may provide chemotherapy prior to transplant and help treat the side effects associated with the medication. Because recovery after BMT is extensive, these nurses also help manage symptoms and treatment in the following months. These nurses must be specially trained in dealing with serious health conditions associated with BMT and know how to intervene appropriately in emergencies.

EDUCATIONAL REQUIREMENTS

RN preparation is required. Certification as Blood & Marrow Transplant Certified Nurse through the Oncology Nursing Certification Corporation is encouraged.

CORE COMPETENCIES/SKILLS NEEDED

- Certification in chemotherapy
- Strong knowledge of pathophysiology about cancers that affect blood and bone marrow
- Competency in intravenous skills including starting, maintaining, and troubleshooting related problems
- Ability to manage patients experiencing an oncologic emergency
- Good interpersonal and communication skills
- Ability to maintain levelheadedness during times of stress
- Knowledge of the BMT procedure

RELATED WEBSITES AND PROFESSIONAL ORGANIZATIONS

- Educational Material (www.bmtcare.com)
- Oncology Nursing Certification Corporation (www.oncc.org)
- Oncology Nursing Society (www.ons.org)

27 BONE MARROW TRANSPLANT NURSE PRACTITIONER

BASIC DESCRIPTION

Bone marrow transplant (BMT) nurse practitioners are advanced practice nurses who provide collaborative care for patients who have or will receive a BMT secondary to cancer, anemia, or other bone marrow disorders. They are responsible for obtaining a thorough history and physical of their patients, ordering and interpreting relevant diagnostic laboratory and imaging tests, and developing and individualizing treatment plans. BMT nurse practitioners can work in inpatient hospital settings, or also in outpatient clinics or infusion treatment areas, and can follow their patients throughout their course of treatment and recovery.

EDUCATIONAL REQUIREMENTS

RN preparation is required. A Master of Science in Nursing (MSN) with advanced practice certification as a nurse practitioner is required. Certification is available through the American Association of Nurse Practitioners and American Nurses Credentialing Center. Basic life support and advanced cardiac life support certifications are also necessary. Certification for Advanced Oncology Certified Nurse Practitioner is encouraged.

CORE COMPETENCIES/SKILLS NEEDED
- Ability to work as part of a team
- Excellent assessment, communication, and critical thinking skills
- Extensive knowledge of diseases of bone marrow and BMT procedure
- Excellent communication and organizational skills

RELATED WEBSITES AND PROFESSIONAL ORGANIZATIONS
- American Association of Nurse Practitioners (www.aanp.org)
- American Nurses Credentialing Center (www.nursecredentialing.org)
- Educational Material (www.bmtcare.com)
- Oncology Nursing Certification Corporation (www.oncc.org)
- Oncology Nursing Society (www.ons.org)

BREAST CARE NURSE **28**

BASIC DESCRIPTION
Breast care nurses specialize in caring for patients diagnosed with breast cancer. They provide holistic nursing care that involves assessing breast cancer risks, providing treatment based on a physician's directives, and educating patients with regard to symptom management, psychosocial and spiritual support, and end-of-life care.

EDUCATIONAL REQUIREMENTS
RN preparation is required; certification is offered by the Oncology Nursing Certification Corporation.

CORE COMPETENCIES/SKILLS NEEDED
- Excellent communication skills
- Ability to provide sensitive care to patients and their families
- Knowledge of resources and agencies for breast cancer patients and survivors
- Knowledge of palliative and end-of-life care
- Knowledge of evidence-based information on breast cancer prevention, care, and management

RELATED WEBSITES AND PROFESSIONAL ORGANIZATIONS
- National Breast Cancer Foundation, Inc. (www.nationalbreastcancer.org)
- Oncology Nursing Certification Corporation (www.oncc.org/TakeTest/Certifications/CBCN)
- The Breast Cancer Site (www.thebreastcancersite.com/clickToGive/home.faces?siteId=2)

29 BURN NURSE

BASIC DESCRIPTION

Nurses who work with burn patients perform comprehensive, highly specialized critical care to adult, geriatric, and pediatric patients who have sustained burn injuries involving up to 100% of total body surface area. The working environment on a burn unit is very intense. The nurse must continually be involved in assessment, planning, and evaluation of care. As part of a highly functioning interdisciplinary team, the nurse must recognize physiological and behavioral changes and know their significance to patient survival. Burn nurses administer pain and other medications, operate special equipment specific to the burn unit, and must maintain fluid and electrolyte balance in their patients.

EDUCATIONAL REQUIREMENTS

RN preparation is required.

CORE COMPETENCIES/SKILLS NEEDED

Most burn units require 1 year of general medical–surgical or critical care experience, as well as the following:

- Knowledge of the pathophysiology of burns
- Complete understanding of fluid and electrolyte balance
- Technical competency involving complex equipment
- Ability to work with patients on ventilators
- Knowledge of pain management
- Skill in the use of aseptic technique
- Interpersonal competency dealing with patients and families in life-threatening situations
- Ability to work with interdisciplinary teams

RELATED WEBSITES AND PROFESSIONAL ORGANIZATIONS

- American Burn Association (www.ameriburn.org)
- Nurse Friendly (www.nursefriendly.com/burn)

BURN NURSE PRACTITIONER

BASIC DESCRIPTION
A burn treatment nurse practitioner assesses, manages, and evaluates the care of patients in a burn unit. Other responsibilities include health teaching, discharge planning, and coordination of care of patients in a burn unit. Administrative responsibilities include participation in research activities, providing training and lectures at partner institutions or community groups, and participating in quality improvement projects or activities.

EDUCATIONAL REQUIREMENTS
RN preparation and nurse practitioner certification are required; at least 2 to 3 years of acute care experience preferably in an intensive care unit (ICU) is highly desired in most positions; Advanced Burn Life Support course is available from the American Burn Association.

CORE COMPETENCIES/SKILLS NEEDED
- Excellent assessment and critical analysis skills
- Excellent interpersonal and communication skills
- Sensitivity to the needs of patients and their families
- Advanced knowledge and training in burn and pain management
- Ability to work in a team
- Leadership and organizational skills
- Ability to identify and intervene when critical deviations in patient conditions are noted

RELATED WEBSITES AND PROFESSIONAL ORGANIZATIONS
- American Burn Association (www.ameriburn.org)
- Burn Prevention Network (www.burnprevention.org)
- Canadian Association of Burn Nurses (www.cabn.ca/E-main.php)

31

BUSINESS OWNER

BASIC DESCRIPTION

A business owner is someone who owns and cultivates a business. The business can be related in any way to the health care industry. Examples include corporations and industry, private practices, devices used in health care, or any type of health care facility. The business owner may be an entrepreneur who created the business or may have acquired the business through other means.

EDUCATION REQUIREMENTS

A bachelor's degree in a health care–related field and/or business is desirable. A master's degree is preferred.

CORE COMPETENCIES/SKILLS NEEDED

- Problem-solving skills
- Creativity and flexibility
- Self-motivation, ambition, and determination
- Willingness to take risks and make important decisions
- Ability to work independently
- Excellent leadership and communication skills
- Knowledge of finance and business
- Desire to work independently

RELATED WEBSITES AND PROFESSIONAL ORGANIZATIONS

- National Nurses in Business Association (www.nnbanow.com)
- U.S. Small Business Administration (www.sba.gov)

CAMP NURSE

BASIC DESCRIPTION

A camp nurse provides full health care to children attending camp. In some situations, camps are specific to children with special needs, for example, children with asthma, or children with diabetes. The working environment for a camp nurse is usually one of low stress. Much of the time is spent working with groups of children in an outdoor setting. The work is normally short term during the summer months. However, if a crisis arises, the nurse must have the critical care and rapid response background to deal with life-threatening situations.

EDUCATIONAL REQUIREMENTS

RN preparation is required.

CORE COMPETENCIES/SKILLS NEEDED

Camp nurses require knowledge of first aid, cardiopulmonary resuscitation (CPR), bee stings, snakebites, cuts, and other acute traumatic episodes. Other requirements include the following:

- Understanding separation anxiety
- Interpersonal skills
- First aid knowledge
- Physical and emotional assessment skills
- Medication management
- Ability to respond to unexpected situations

RELATED WEBSITES AND PROFESSIONAL ORGANIZATIONS

- Association of Camp Nurses (www.campnurse.org)
- Camp Nurse Jobs (www.campnursejobs.com)

33 CARDIAC CATHETERIZATION NURSE

BASIC DESCRIPTION
A cardiac catheterization nurse has a specialized role and is a highly skilled cardiovascular nurse whose primary responsibility includes providing nursing care for patients undergoing cardiac catheterization. The spectrum of responsibilities ranges from preadmission to discharge that could include conducting a health screen, preparing patients before the surgery, assisting the surgeon during the surgical procedure, monitoring patients after the surgery, and discharging patients.

EDUCATIONAL REQUIREMENTS
RN preparation and at least 1 year of critical care or emergency room experience are preferred; advanced cardiac life support and basic life support certifications are required; critical care registered nurse (CCRN) and/or registered cardiovascular invasive specialist certification are highly desirable.

CORE COMPETENCIES/SKILLS NEEDED
- Excellent communication skills
- Knowledge of cardiovascular physiology and pathophysiology and cardiac dysrhythmias and their interventions
- Ability to wear lead protection while at work

RELATED WEBSITES AND PROFESSIONAL ORGANIZATIONS
- American Association of Critical-Care Nurses (www.aacn.org)
- Cardiovascular Credentialing International (www.cci-online.org)

CARDIOPULMONARY RESUSCITATION INSTRUCTOR

34

BASIC DESCRIPTION

Cardiopulmonary resuscitation (CPR) nursing instructors are nurses who have undergone special training to teach and certify people in CPR. Audiences for CPR training can be coworkers, friends and family, volunteers, members of the community, or medical professionals. It is the responsibility of the instructor to ensure that the trainees have the knowledge and skills necessary to perform effective CPR in emergent situations. They are also responsible for ensuring that the trainees receive their certification after training through the certifying organization.

EDUCATION REQUIREMENTS

RN preparation and certification in CPR are essential prior to instructor training. Successful completion of instructor training through the certification organization is required. Some requirements for instructor certification and certification renewal vary, depending on the organization through which one becomes a certified CPR instructor.

CORE COMPETENCIES/SKILLS NEEDED

- Effective communication skills
- Ability to teach and remediate skills
- Basic computer skills
- Understanding of CPR skills and rationale
- Knowledge of certification process

RELATED WEBSITES AND PROFESSIONAL ORGANIZATIONS

- American Heart Association (www.heart.org)
- American Red Cross (www.redcross.org)
- National Safety Council (www.nsc.org)

35 CARDIOTHORACIC INTENSIVE CARE NURSE

BASIC DESCRIPTION
A cardiothoracic intensive care nurse works in a highly specialized cardiothoracic intensive care unit (ICU) catering to the needs of patients requiring constant monitoring and whose clinical conditions are considered critical. The cardiothoracic intensive care nurse is adept at noting subtle hemodynamic changes that could lead to serious complications and providing immediate interventions as required. The ICU nurse is comfortable in operating and managing complex medical equipment such as ventilators and telemetry monitors and works closely with physicians and unlicensed assistive personnel. The cardiothoracic intensive care nurse usually takes care of no more than two acutely ill patients in a shift.

EDUCATIONAL REQUIREMENTS
RN preparation, basic life support certification, and advanced cardiac life support certification are required; certification as a critical care registered nurse is available from the American Association of Critical-Care Nurses.

CORE COMPETENCIES/SKILLS NEEDED
- Ability to work in a dynamic and intense environment that requires quick thinking and excellent analytical and assessment skills
- Strong background knowledge on hemodynamics, arrhythmia management, pathophysiology, and pharmacology
- Excellent interpersonal and communication skills
- Excellent technical skills such as intravenous management and ventilator care
- Strong computer skills needed for electronic health record documentation
- Strong leadership and delegation skills

RELATED WEBSITES AND PROFESSIONAL ORGANIZATION
- American Association of Critical-Care Nurses (www.aacn.org)
- American Nurses Credentialing Center (www.nursecredentialing.org)

CARDIOTHORACIC INTENSIVE CARE NURSE PRACTITIONER

36

BASIC DESCRIPTION
A cardiothoracic intensive care nurse practitioner provides primary care to adults who have acute and complex cardiovascular conditions that require constant monitoring. The cardiothoracic intensive care nurse practitioner works in a highly specialized acute care unit that caters to the needs of patients who have undergone coronary artery bypass graft surgery, heart valve replacement, pacemaker and internal defibrillator placement, heart and lung transplants, and other major cardiothoracic surgeries.

EDUCATIONAL REQUIREMENTS
RN preparation and nurse practitioner certification, master's degree in nursing or higher, and basic life support and advanced cardiac life support certifications are required. Certification as acute care nurse practitioner is offered by the American Association of Critical-Care Nurses and American Nurses Credentialing Center.

CORE COMPETENCIES/SKILLS NEEDED
- Excellent assessment and decision-making skills
- Advanced knowledge in hemodynamic pathophysiology, assessment, diagnosis, management, and pharmacology
- Strong leadership and organizational skills
- A high level of stress tolerance and the ability to work in fast-paced and highly dynamic environments
- Ability to work autonomously
- Possible involvement in unit- or hospital-based clinical research

RELATED WEBSITES AND PROFESSIONAL ORGANIZATIONS
- American Association of Critical-Care Nurses (www.aacn.org)
- American Nurses Credentialing Center (www.nursecredentialing.org)

37 CARDIOTHORACIC NURSE ANESTHETIST

BASIC DESCRIPTION

A cardiothoracic nurse anesthetist works in collaboration with anesthesiologists to provide anesthesia care to patients undergoing heart transplants, ventricular remodeling, and cardiothoracic operations.

EDUCATIONAL REQUIREMENTS

RN preparation and certification as a certified registered nurse anesthetist are required; basic life support and advanced cardiac life support certifications are also required. Experience in acute or emergency care is required as a prerequisite to most positions; certification is offered by the National Board of Certification & Recertification of Nurse Anesthetists.

CORE COMPETENCIES/SKILLS NEEDED

- Excellent interpersonal and communication skills
- Excellent assessment skills and advanced knowledge in cardiovascular, pulmonary, and hemodynamic physiology, management, and pharmacology
- Ability to work in a high-stress environment that requires quick decision making
- Strong computer and documentation skills and knowledge of electronic health record

RELATED WEBSITES AND PROFESSIONAL ORGANIZATIONS

- American Association of Nurse Anesthetists (www.aana.com)
- International Federation of Nurse Anesthetists (ifna-int.org/ifna/news.php)
- National Board of Certification & Recertification of Nurse Anesthetists (www.nbcrna.com)

CARDIOVASCULAR NURSE

BASIC DESCRIPTION

The cardiovascular nurse works with patients who have a compromised cardiovascular system. Cardiac nurses perform postoperative care on a surgical unit, stress test evaluations, cardiac monitoring, vascular monitoring, and health assessments. The setting can be varied depending on the focus of the patient population. Cardiovascular nurses can work in acute care settings with surgical patients, in outpatient clinics doing case management, and in home care.

EDUCATIONAL REQUIREMENTS

RN preparation and basic life support and advanced cardiac life support certifications are required. Certification as a cardiovascular nurse is available from the American Nurses Credentialing Center and as a critical care nurse from the American Association of Critical-Care Nurses.

CORE COMPETENCIES/SKILLS NEEDED

- Proficiency in reading cardiac monitors
- Critical care experience
- Knowledge of cardiac rhythms and cardiac disease
- Good interpersonal skills
- Ability to work with interdisciplinary teams
- Ability to manage acute episodes in chronically ill patients

RELATED WEBSITES AND PROFESSIONAL ORGANIZATIONS

- American Association of Cardiovascular and Pulmonary Rehabilitation (www.aacvpr.org)
- Association for Vascular Access (www.avainfo.org)
- Society for Vascular Nursing (www.svnnet.org)

39

CARE COORDINATOR

BASIC DESCRIPTION
A nurse who works as a care coordinator oversees a patient's care. He or she focuses on helping patients navigate the health care system efficiently and easily to improve or maintain optimal health. These nurses coordinate and collaborate with other health care providers to ensure quality care and adequate follow-up visits to promote the highest possible quality of life. Care coordinators also provide patients and their families with personalized plans and the resources they need to participate in care and ensure best outcomes.

EDUCATION REQUIREMENTS
Preparation as an RN is required. Relevant nursing experience is recommended.

CORE COMPETENCIES/SKILLS NEEDED
- Organization and coordination skills
- Ability to collaborate with multiple health care professionals and also work independently
- Strong communication skills
- Excellent problem-solving skills
- Ability to educate patients and families about health care plans

RELATED WEBSITE AND PROFESSIONAL ORGANIZATION
- American Nurses Association (www.ana.org)

CASE MANAGER

BASIC DESCRIPTION
Case management is the process of organizing and coordinating resources and services in response to individual health care needs along the illness and care continuum in multiple settings. There are many models for case management based on client, context, or setting. The nurse case manager assesses and monitors clients and the health care delivery services that they require. Case management is directed toward a targeted or selected client/family population, such as transplant, head-injured, or frail elderly clients. The goals are to center services around the patient, to foster patient self-managed care, and to maximize efficient and cost-effective use of health resources. The focus is cost saving and continuity of care. Case managers have the opportunity to work in hospitals, community outreach clinics, occupational health, insurance companies, and health maintenance organizations.

EDUCATIONAL REQUIREMENTS
RN preparation and Bachelor of Science in Nursing are required; a master's degree is preferred. Certification in case management is available from the American Nurses Credentialing Center.

CORE COMPETENCIES/SKILLS NEEDED
- Strong knowledge base in both the financial and clinical aspects of care
- Understanding of community resources
- Strong communication skills
- Effective skills in managing, teaching, and negotiating
- Ability to work with interdisciplinary groups
- Ability to focus on patients and families

RELATED WEBSITES AND PROFESSIONAL ORGANIZATIONS
- American Association of Managed Care Nurses (www.aamcn.org)
- American Nurses Credentialing Center (www.nursecredentialing.org)
- Case Management Society of America (www.cmsa.org)
- Commission for Case Manager Certification (www.ccmcertification.org)

41 CENTRAL INTELLIGENCE AGENCY OCCUPATIONAL HEALTH NURSE

BASIC DESCRIPTION
A Central Intelligence Agency (CIA) occupational health nurse is responsible for addressing health concerns of CIA employees in the workplace. They work to implement interventions to prevent workplace health problems, and to assess and treat or refer occupation-related health complaints. They also may perform basic health screenings.

EDUCATION REQUIREMENTS
RN preparation with a bachelor's degree in nursing is required. Experience as a critical, emergency, or occupational health nurse is also required.

CORE COMPETENCIES/SKILLS REQUIRED
- Knowledge of first aid
- Experience in emergency, critical, or occupational care
- Requirement to pass background check, polygraph test, medical exam, and psychological exam
- Self-discipline
- Ability to maintain discretion
- Good assessment and documentation skills
- Knowledge of potential workplace hazards and effective prevention or treatment strategies
- Ability to educate patients on workplace hazards

RELATED WEBSITES AND PROFESSIONAL ORGANIZATIONS
- American Board of Occupational Health Nurses, Inc. (www.abohn.org)
- Central Intelligence Agency (www.CIA.gov)
- Occupational Safety and Health Administration (www.osha.gov)

CERTIFIED REGISTERED NURSE ANESTHETIST

BASIC DESCRIPTION
Certified registered nurse anesthetists (CRNAs) are advanced practice nurses who provide anesthesia care to patients, often in collaboration with surgeons, anesthesiologists, dentists, and other health care professionals. They work with a high level of autonomy and responsibility. Anesthesia administered by a CRNA compared to that by an anesthesiologist is the same; the difference is the practice by which it is given (nursing versus medicine). In addition to administering anesthesia, CRNAs are responsible for completing a preanesthetic assessment, maintaining patient safety while under anesthesia, and managing the patient after discontinuation of anesthesia. CRNAs can work wherever anesthesia is administered: operating rooms in a hospital, ambulatory surgery centers, obstetrical delivery rooms, dentist offices, and more.

EDUCATIONAL REQUIREMENTS
RN preparation and graduation from an accredited master's level nurse anesthesia program are both required. Passing the National Certification Exam by the National Board of Certification & Recertification of Nurse Anesthetists after graduation is essential. Nurses also need at least 1 year of clinical experience in an intensive care setting, such as an intensive care unit, prior to entering a graduate in nurse anesthesia program. Basic life support and advanced cardiac life support certification are also required.

CORE COMPETENCIES/SKILLS NEEDED
- Critical thinking skills
- Thorough knowledge of medications administered by CRNAs
- Ability to make important decisions quickly under stress
- Strong computer and documentation skills
- Excellent communication skills
- Excellent assessment skills and advanced knowledge of anatomy, physiology, pathophysiology, and pharmacology

RELATED WEBSITES AND PROFESSIONAL ORGANIZATIONS
- American Association of Nurse Anesthetists (www.aana.com)
- International Federation of Nurse Anesthetists (ifna.site)
- National Board of Certification & Recertification of Nurse Anesthetists (www.nbcrna.com)

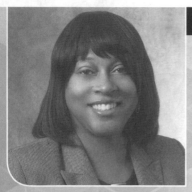

 PROFILE: **SONYA D. MOORE**
Nurse Anesthesia Program Director

1. What is your educational background in nursing (and other areas) and what formal credentials do you hold?

I am the director of a nurse anesthesia program at a prominent, private, nonprofit university. Alongside my appointment of instructor, I have held the program director's position for 2 years, and previously I was the assistant program director and clinical coordinator. I have 20 years of experience as a CRNA, 10 of them in my own practice. My credentials include a Bachelor of Science in Nursing, a Master of Science in Nursing, and a Doctorate of Nursing Practice.

2. How did you first become interested in your current career?

I first became interested in nurse anesthesia through a high school program in which participants had the opportunity to shadow medical professionals. This was a critical moment for me. It was then that I became aware of career paths I might never have known about as a student in an inner-city school system. From that point, I began the process of researching this professional pathway and aligning it to my personal goals. Shadowing showed me I could get there; all I had to do was figure out how.

3. What are the most rewarding aspects of your career?

As a nurse educator, I am always pleased to see others step forward to take on the mantle of my profession. I feel strongly about mentoring, because some form of that got me where I am today. Seeking to become an advanced practice nurse can present its own burden to my students, but that is exactly where my role activates best in assisting and encouraging

Continued

them while they learn to "shift the weight" and keep standing. I myself must be an example administratively and professionally, and it is most rewarding when students of mine who have graduated honor me by calling me their colleague.

4. What advice would you give to someone contemplating the same career path in nursing?

Plan and persevere—quite simple instructions that are indeed hard to follow, but that is exactly what it takes to make it through both training and professional hurdles. A general perception of my profession is that it is easy in comparison to more noticeably physical practices. As a nurse anesthetist, one's mind must be alert and focused on a singular-entwined task for long stretches of time—keeping someone alive. Airway, hemodynamics, consciousness, drug interactions, position, heart rate, temperature, body size, health condition, time . . . I must consider and be aware of all of these while poised, watching the breaths of patients who may meet me for only a few minutes before sleeping for hours, hoping to wake up better than when they lay down.

43 CHEMOTHERAPY NURSE

BASIC DESCRIPTION
Chemotherapy nursing is a specialty within oncology nursing. Chemotherapy nurses administer and monitor the patient receiving chemotherapeutic agents as ordered by physicians. Working closely with oncologists and pharmacists, chemotherapy nurses' job responsibilities could also include obtaining patient histories, collecting specimens, evaluating effectiveness of treatment, and educating patients on treatment and follow-up care.

EDUCATIONAL REQUIREMENTS
RN preparation is required, and a Bachelor of Science in Nursing is preferred. Basic life support certification is required, and advanced cardiac life support certification is preferred; certification as an oncology certified nurse could be obtained by passing a certification examination offered by the Oncology Nursing Society's Oncology Nursing Certification Corporation. For recertification, 1,000 hours of clinical practice in oncology and continuing professional development activities are required.

CORE COMPETENCIES/SKILLS NEEDED
- Excellent intravenous skills including starting, maintaining, and troubleshooting common intravenous access problems
- Excellent communication skills and organizational skills
- Knowledge of cancer, its pathophysiology, and common treatments and side effects

RELATED WEBSITES AND PROFESSIONAL ORGANIZATIONS
- Association of Pediatric Hematology/Oncology Nurses (www.aphon.org)
- Oncology Nursing Society (www.ons.org)

CHIEF LEARNING OFFICER

BASIC DESCRIPTION

A chief learning officer is a nursing leader who is an expert in and manages the learning environment in a health care setting. A chief learning officer will work with the chief executive officer (CEO) to ensure goals of the organization are met through educational advancement and learning-based initiatives. Employment can be found in an academic or health care setting.

EDUCATIONAL REQUIREMENTS

RN preparation is required. A Bachelor of Science in Nursing and a master's degree in nursing or education is necessary. Doctorate level of education or MBA is also highly desirable.

CORE COMPETENCIES/SKILLS NEEDED

- Excellent leadership and management skills
- Ability to collaborate
- Motivational and mentoring skills
- Ability to make sound decisions
- Skills in education, learning theory, technology, and management
- Ability to inspire others
- Research and publication skills

RELATED WEBSITES AND PROFESSIONAL ORGANIZATIONS

- American Association of Colleges of Nursing (www.aacn.nche.edu)
- National League for Nursing (www.nln.org)

45 CHIEF NURSING INFORMATION OFFICER

BASIC DESCRIPTION
A chief nursing information officer is a nurse in a leadership role that incorporates nursing science and health information technology and applies this knowledge to nursing practice and health care delivery. Employment opportunities can be found in a health care system, information technology companies, or in the government and nursing organizations.

EDUCATIONAL REQUIREMENTS
RN preparation with a master's degree in nursing informatics is required. Credentialing is available through the American Nurses Credentialing Center.

CORE COMPETENCIES/SKILLS NEEDED
- Ability to conduct information analyses and develop data analysis systems and methodologies
- Consultation skills regarding the use of technology
- Marketing skills
- Skill in developing and disseminating reports to staff about cost and other trends in health care
- Strong organizational skills
- Ability to use various resources to analyze and interpret variances and make comparisons with national and regional benchmarks
- Excellent professional, leadership, and management skills
- Creativity and ability to solve problems
- Ability to be objective and assertive
- Strong communication and interpersonal skills
- Ability to collaborate and work well with a team

RELATED WEBSITES AND PROFESSIONAL ORGANIZATIONS
- American Medical Informatics Association: Nursing Informatics Working Group (www.amia.org/programs/working-groups/nursing-informatics)
- American Nurses Credentialing Center (www.ancc.org)
- American Nursing Informatics Association (www.ania.org)

CHIEF NURSING OFFICER 46

BASIC DESCRIPTION
A chief nursing officer is the executive nurse leader of a health care organization. He or she connects clinical and business operations and is ultimately responsible for all nursing-related operations in the hospital setting, including patient satisfaction, financial planning, clinical skills, organizational compliance, regulatory standards, and quality improvement.

EDUCATIONAL REQUIREMENTS
RN preparation is required. Experience in a nursing leadership position with a master's degree in nursing is required. A doctorate in nursing or a related field is highly desirable. Certification is available through the American Nurses Credentialing Center.

CORE COMPETENCIES/SKILLS NEEDED
- Excellent leadership and management skills
- Ability to be assertive, objective, and make important decisions under pressure
- Strong communication and interpersonal skills
- Willingness to take risks
- Business knowledge and financial skills
- Ability to work independently or collaboratively with multiple departments and disciplines
- Skills in using technology
- Understanding of budgeting and finance
- Strong clinical skills

RELATED WEBSITES AND PROFESSIONAL ORGANIZATIONS
- American College of Healthcare Executives (www.ache.org)
- American Nurses Credentialing Center (www.nursecredentialing.org)
- American Organization of Nurse Executives (www.aone.org)

47 CHILD–ADOLESCENT PSYCHIATRIC–MENTAL HEALTH CLINICAL NURSE SPECIALIST

BASIC DESCRIPTION
A child–adolescent psychiatric–mental health clinical nurse specialist (CNS) is an advanced practice nurse who works with children and adolescents with psychiatric problems, focusing on the individual client/patient with any presenting health problem. The advanced practice role is aimed at early intervention and treatment of children with mental illness, and includes use of a wide range of psychotherapeutic skills (e.g., individual, family, and group therapy). The child–adolescent psychiatric–mental health CNS practices in both inpatient and outpatient hospital settings and a variety of other settings such as clinics, schools, community agencies, day treatment facilities, and public health departments. Additional advanced practice activities include consultation with other professional and nonprofessional groups and education of other professionals, administrators, and researchers.

EDUCATIONAL REQUIREMENTS
RN preparation and licensure, advanced practice licensure, and master's, post-master's, or doctoral preparation in a CNS program in child–adolescent psychiatric–mental health nursing are required. Advanced practice certification requires a minimum of 500 supervised clinical hours in the specialty. Certification from the American Nurses Credentialing Center is available.

CORE COMPETENCIES/SKILLS NEEDED
- Advanced assessment skills
- Advanced knowledge of pharmacology and pathophysiology
- Ability to meet the child at his or her developmental level
- Clinical skill in at least two psychotherapeutic treatment modalities
- Ability to facilitate coordination and collaboration among agencies delivering care to children
- Ability to provide services to children and their families
- Flexibility and sensitivity

RELATED WEBSITES AND PROFESSIONAL ORGANIZATIONS
- American Nurses Credentialing Center (www.nursecredentialing.org)
- American Psychiatric Nurses Association (www.apna.org)
- Association of Child and Adolescent Psychiatric Nurses Division, International Society of Psychiatric–Mental Health Nurses (www.ispn-psych .org)

CHILDBIRTH EDUCATOR

48

BASIC DESCRIPTION
The childbirth educator provides informational and educational classes for expectant parents. Classes include information on relaxation techniques, comfort measures, breathing techniques, and birth options. Childbirth educators play an important role in the emotional, physical, and informational support for expectant parents. Most hospitals and birthing centers offer this type of educational program for their clients. Usually, a nurse with excellent teaching and interpersonal skills is selected to teach class on site.

EDUCATIONAL REQUIREMENTS
RN preparation is required. A certification may be obtained through the Childbirth and Postpartum Professional Association.

CORE COMPETENCIES/SKILLS NEEDED
- Knowledge about the childbearing years, pregnancy, and labor and delivery
- Teaching ability
- Clinical competence in obstetrical nursing
- Interpersonal skills
- Ability to collaborate with physicians

RELATED WEBSITES AND PROFESSIONAL ORGANIZATIONS
- Childbirth and Postpartum Professional Association (www.cappa.net)
- Childbirth.org (www.childbirth.org)
- Lamaze International (www.lamaze.com)

49 CHILD PSYCHIATRIC NURSE

BASIC DESCRIPTION
A child psychiatric nurse is one who works with children and adolescents with psychiatric problems, and who focuses on the entire continuum between health and illness. The nurse's role is aimed at promotion and prevention, early intervention, and treatment of children with mental illness. The child psychiatric nurse practices in a variety of settings such as clinics, schools, community agencies, psychiatric hospitals, day treatment facilities, and public health departments. Generalist activities of a child psychiatric nurse include teaching parents with emotionally disturbed or mentally challenged children or adolescents, participation as a member of a health care delivery team, and participation in research activities related to the field of child and adolescent psychiatric nursing.

EDUCATIONAL REQUIREMENTS
RN preparation and licensure, with certification in psychiatric–mental health nursing, are required.

CORE COMPETENCIES/SKILLS NEEDED
- Ability to meet the child at his or her developmental level
- Knowledgeable about psychiatric mental health treatment and services
- Ability to facilitate coordination and collaboration among agencies delivering care to children
- Ability to provide services to children and their families
- Flexibility and sensitivity

RELATED WEBSITES AND PROFESSIONAL ORGANIZATIONS
- American Nurses Credentialing Center (www.nursecredentialing.org)
- American Psychiatric Nurses Association (www.apna.org)

CIRCULATING NURSE

BASIC DESCRIPTION
The circulating nurse, an integral part of the perioperative team, serves as an advocate for patients who are under anesthesia and/or sedation. Responsibilities include ensuring that surgical asepsis is adhered to during the surgical procedure, keeping track and conducting an inventory of supplies and equipment used during and after the surgical procedure, or calling for a time out. The Joint Commission has specified a "time out" immediately before surgery to prevent surgical errors.

EDUCATIONAL REQUIREMENTS
RN preparation is required. Advanced cardiac life support and basic life support certifications are mostly required for this position. Nurse operating room certification is highly desirable.

CORE COMPETENCIES/SKILLS NEEDED
- Excellent communication skills
- Ability to work with members of the perioperative team
- Excellent observation skills
- Knowledge of asepsis, infection control, and effects of anesthesia

RELATED WEBSITES AND PROFESSIONAL ORGANIZATIONS
- Association of periOperative Registered Nurses (www.aorn.org)
- Competency and Credentialing Institute (www.cc-institute.org)

51

CLINICAL/DRUG SAFETY ASSOCIATE

BASIC DESCRIPTION
A clinical safety associate or drug safety associate works as part of the pharmaceutical industry by studying and delivering information regarding medication safety and medication management. Nurses in this position work to perform quality reviews and ensure proper regulatory reporting and compliance with regards to drug safety.

EDUCATION REQUIREMENTS
A bachelor's degree in nursing or a health care–related field is required with relevant clinical experience.

CORE COMPETENCIES/SKILLS NEEDED
- Ability to pay attention to quality and detail
- Ability to analyze and synthesize data
- Knowledge of adverse event coding systems
- Understanding of United States and European Union safety regulations
- Problem-solving skills
- Knowledge of pharmaceutical products
- Excellent oral and written communication skills

RELATED WEBSITES AND PROFESSIONAL ORGANIZATIONS
- Pharmaceutical Representatives Online (www.pharmrep.com)
- Pharmaceutical Research and Manufacturers of America (www.phrma.org)

CLINICAL EDUCATOR/DIRECTOR

52

BASIC DESCRIPTION

A clinical educator/director is a leader who works with departmental directors to ensure educational goals are met. The director will delegate tasks and initiatives to educators to ensure that nurses are gaining the knowledge they need to develop professionally and improve their practice. The director is responsible for the coordination of educational initiatives and their dissemination to the appropriate departments in a timely fashion. Employment is typically found in a hospital or health care system. The director of education may also play a role in development or revision of institutional policies and procedures.

EDUCATIONAL REQUIREMENTS

RN preparation is required. A master's degree in nursing or education is also necessary. Previous experience in education is highly desirable. Certification is also available.

CORE COMPETENCIES/SKILLS NEEDED

- Highly motivated and organized
- Motivational and mentoring skills
- Ability to collaborate and delegate
- Computer and technological skills
- Knowledge of learning theories and principles
- Knowledge of teaching/learning and/or management principles and practices
- Ability to make sound decisions
- Research and publication skills
- Excellent communication and interpersonal skills

RELATED WEBSITES AND PROFESSIONAL ORGANIZATIONS

- American Association of Colleges of Nursing (www.aacn.nche.edu)
- National League for Nursing (www.nln.org)

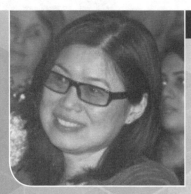

 PROFILE: **JENNY XIANG**

Nurse Educator, Clinical Setting

1. What is your educational background in nursing (and other areas) and what formal credentials do you hold?

I came to the United States in 1986. I received my associate degree while working as a companion at night. Then I obtained a Bachelor of Science in Nursing (BSN) degree while working as a staff nurse full time. From there, I continued my education and received a master's degree in nursing education with a focus on adult learning. I have certifications in both critical care and medical–surgical nursing. I hope to become a nursing professional development specialist by the end of the year.

2. How did you first become interested in the career that you are currently in?

My interest in nursing education started during my preceptorship as a new graduate nurse in the intensive care unit (ICU) while working as a clinical nurse. Traditionally a new graduate nurse must work in the medical–surgical unit for 2 years before going to any specialty area. I have always been a person who loves mentoring, teaching, and keeping up with technology that can help us in the nursing field. Soon after, I found a part-time position as a clinical instructor. I am very thankful for that position; I gained many memories and was proud to be a teacher. One day I received a letter from one of my nursing students, who wrote: "As my first clinical instructor, you taught me the value of relentlessness and confidence. I am grateful to you for my career as a nurse."

After working as a bedside nurse in the ICU full time for 22 years and teaching as a clinical instructor part time for 5 years, I decided to pursue a full-time job in nursing education. I was fortunate to be hired as a nurse educator when the health system for which I work decided to open a sixth location in downtown New York City, and a position opened up. Since starting here, I have helped to implement a number of programs, including

Continued

a General Nursing Orientation program, Preceptor workshop, Charge Nurse workshop, Crisis Prevention Intervention program, Hospital Infection Prevention program, and Operating Room New Graduate Nurses program. As a nurse educator, I feel like I am on stage every day when I am either teaching or making rounds of the units. I am not only a resource person, but also someone with whom other staff can talk, whether about a rough day at work or the decision to go back to school, transfer to a specialty area, or become certified in their practice area.

3. What are the most rewarding aspects of your career?

My job is unique on many levels. I love to meet newly hired nurses every month and give them advice as many are just beginning their nursing professional careers. Over the past 2 1/2 years, the organization where I work has undergone tremendous changes, including a new leadership team, endless new equipment training and computer upgrades, opening of a new unit, and expansion of the old unit. The most rewarding aspect of my career just happened—during 2016 Nurses Week. My dedication to being a nurse educator resonated at the Nursing Excellence Award celebration, when all the award recipients shouted out my name to thank me for being a supportive mentor over time. This small token of recognition from other nurses made me realize the impact that I have had on others, which has been so rewarding throughout my career.

4. What advice would you give to someone contemplating the same career path in nursing?

I would tell new nurses who are just beginning their careers to build a solid foundation in what they want to do in nursing. Each nursing skill, whether it is simple patient assessment, patient care, or patient and family teaching, will help you advance in your future career and can only help you. I would also encourage anyone interested in nursing education to join national professional organizations. New and seasoned nurses should also attend national or worldwide conferences and educational seminars, read journal articles to stay up to date with what is happening, and network. Nursing is a lifelong journey and learning experience. Nursing as a profession is always evolving. The nursing shortage, external regulatory changes, aging baby boomers, and the proliferation of opportunities, both within and beyond the field of nursing, all contribute to the current sense of challenges and possibilities.

53 CLINICAL NURSE SPECIALIST

BASIC DESCRIPTION
A clinical nurse specialist (CNS) coordinates activities regarding patient care on a specific unit within the hospital. The setting is usually inpatient hospital, and intense. CNSs assist the multidisciplinary team from admission to discharge; answer and refer questions the family might have; are involved in health teaching and support/counseling; assist in developing protocols for managing care of the client; serve as resource persons to staff nurses and other health team members; collect data and investigate trends for the program, for example, heart surgery; facilitate discharge preparation for a smooth transmission back home; and coordinate follow-up visits for the patient.

EDUCATIONAL REQUIREMENTS
RN preparation and a Master of Science in Nursing are required. Most settings require 5 years of acute care experience. Certification in various CNS roles is available from the American Association of Critical-Care Nursing and American Nurses Credentialing Center.

CORE COMPETENCIES/SKILLS NEEDED
- Self-confidence and strong leadership skills
- Excellent communication skills
- Understanding of organizational structure
- Technical competency involving use of complex equipment
- Teaching skills
- Clinical competency
- Ability to work with interdisciplinary teams
- Skills in staff evaluation

RELATED WEBSITES AND NURSING ORGANIZATIONS
- American Association of Critical-Care Nurses (www.aacn.org)
- American Board of Nursing Specialties (www.nursingcertification.org)
- American Nurses Credentialing Center (www.nursecredentialing.org)
- National Association of Clinical Nurse Specialists (www.nacns.org)

CLINICAL PROJECT DIRECTOR

BASIC DESCRIPTION

A clinical project director is responsible for the planning, coordination, and execution of clinical projects or clinical trials. He or she is involved from the onset of the project with the proposal and contract development all the way through completion of a project. The project director will collaborate with individuals from appropriate disciplines to ensure proper designs and protocols are carried out. He or she will also develop and follow a plan to manage team members, finances, and scheduling to guarantee smooth functioning of the project.

EDUCATIONAL REQUIREMENTS

RN preparation and a bachelor's degree in nursing are required. A master's degree in nursing or related field is preferred. Project Management Professional certification is highly recommended.

CORE COMPETENCIES/SKILLS NEEDED

- Strong clinical skills and knowledge
- Excellent leadership or management skills
- Highly organized
- Experience or knowledge of finance and budgeting
- Ability to work with a team and collaborate
- Decisiveness and ability to take initiative
- Excellent written and oral communication skills
- Proficiency in computer skills
- Risk assessment and contingency-planning skills
- Thorough knowledge of hospital and regulatory agency policy and protocols
- Knowledge of statistical methods and analyses

RELATED WEBSITES AND PROFESSIONAL ORGANIZATIONS

- National Institute of Nurse Research; a branch of the U.S. Health and Human Services National Institutes of Health (www.ninr.nih.gov)
- National Institutes of Health, Learn About Clinical Trials (clinicaltrials.gov/ct2/info/understand)

55 CLINICAL RESEARCH NURSE

BASIC DESCRIPTION

Clinical research nurses work in clinical research centers and act as patient advocates in ensuring that ethical and efficient care is provided in compliance with federal and local research regulations. Their nursing knowledge provides them with the unique opportunity to meet the complex needs of patients participating in a research study.

EDUCATIONAL REQUIREMENTS

RN preparation, Bachelor of Science in Nursing, and basic life support certification are required. Recent acute care experience is required in most positions.

CORE COMPETENCIES/SKILLS NEEDED

- Knowledge of research process and evidence-based nursing
- Knowledge of institutional review board policies
- Excellent interpersonal and communication skills
- Good computer skills and knowledge of electronic health record

RELATED WEBSITES AND PROFESSIONAL ORGANIZATIONS

- Association of Clinical Research Professionals (www.acrpnet.org)
- Society of Clinical Research Associates (www.socra.org)

COLLEGE/STUDENT HEALTH NURSE PRACTITIONER

56

BASIC DESCRIPTION
College or student health nurse practitioners are advanced practice nurses who deliver care to students at a university, college, or other academic institution. Their practice focuses on health promotion, disease prevention, and crisis intervention. They provide both medical health care and mental health counseling and make appropriate referrals as needed to maintain student health.

EDUCATION REQUIREMENTS
RN preparation is required. A Master of Science in Nursing with advanced practice certification as a nurse practitioner is required. Certification is available through the American Association of Nurse Practitioners and American Nurses Credentialing Center. Basic life support and advanced cardiac life support certifications are also necessary.

CORE COMPETENCIES/SKILLS NEEDED
- Crisis intervention skills
- Knowledge of community resources and ability to make appropriate referrals
- Good communication skills and ability to build relationships with students
- Excellent physical-examination and history-taking skills
- Thorough understanding of communicable diseases
- Ability to assess, diagnose, and treat illness

RELATED WEBSITES AND PROFESSIONAL ORGANIZATIONS
- American Association of Nurse Practitioners (www.aanp.org)
- American Nurses Credentialing Center (www.nursecredentialing.org)

57 COMMUNITY HEALTH NURSE

BASIC DESCRIPTION
A community health nurse is someone who delivers nursing care for individuals and families where they live, work, or go to school. The community health nurse may or may not have education and training in public health nursing. The practice settings for the community health nurse are varied and include home care, school-based care, and occupational health care.

EDUCATIONAL REQUIREMENTS
RN preparation is required and at least 1 year of acute care experience is required for most jobs. Certification is provided by the American Nurses Credentialing Center.

CORE COMPETENCIES/SKILLS NEEDED
- Excellent assessment and communication skills
- Good clinical and analytical skills
- Ability to travel to many locations
- Strong computer skills especially in using portable devices for documentation
- Excellent organization and management skills

RELATED WEBSITES AND PROFESSIONAL ORGANIZATIONS
- American Nurses Credentialing Center (www.nursecredentialing.org)
- American Public Health Association (www.apha.org)
- Association of Community Health Nursing Educators (www.achne.org)

COMPLIANCE SPECIALIST NURSE

BASIC DESCRIPTION
A compliance specialist nurse's primary responsibility is to review medical record claims for a health care organization to assess accuracy of services and quality of care provided, and to assess whether these services have met practice and ethical standard requirements. He or she provides the review team with her clinical expertise in investigating a case.

EDUCATIONAL REQUIREMENTS
RN preparation, Bachelor of Science in Nursing, and at least 3 years of clinical experience, preferably in home care, are desired in most job positions.

CORE COMPETENCIES/SKILLS NEEDED
- Experience in utilization review, risk management, and quality management
- Strong background in clinical compliance, medical record review, and documentation
- Knowledge of Current Procedural Terminology (CPT) and International Classification of Diseases (ICD)-9 codes
- Understanding of Medicare and Medicaid regulations
- Awareness of ethics, ability to be objective, detail oriented, and to work in a high-stress environment
- Strong computer skills and knowledge and data management skills
- Excellent communication, organizational, and interpersonal skills

RELATED WEBSITE AND PROFESSIONAL ORGANIZATION
- Ethics and Compliance Officer Association (ecoaconnects.theecoa.org/home)

59

CONCIERGE NURSE

BASIC DESCRIPTION
A concierge nurse is an RN who assists patients and caregivers with personalized, one-on-one navigation of the health care system. He or she provides support for care management to serve patients by, including but not limited to, locating a health care provider or a specialist, providing education regarding medical diagnoses and treatments, explaining insurance benefits, making or expediting appointments, assisting with referrals, coordinating care, preparing patients for appointments and answering health care–related questions. Job opportunities may be found in private practices, with insurance companies, or in independent concierge service companies.

EDUCATION REQUIREMENTS
RN preparation is required. A bachelor's degree in nursing is preferred. Relevant clinical experience is also required.

CORE COMPETENCIES/SKILLS NEEDED
- Excellent customer service skills
- Effective oral communication
- Strong computer skills
- Empathy and patience
- Excellent clinical judgment
- Systematic problem-solving skills

RELATED WEBSITES AND PROFESSIONAL ORGANIZATIONS
There are no related websites or organizations.

CONCIERGE NURSE PRACTITIONER

60

BASIC DESCRIPTION

With the ever-changing face of health care, new models are emerging for care delivery, including the concept of concierge medicine. With this model, a physician charges a patient an annual fee in exchange for personalized health care services such as house calls, same-day or next-day appointments, 24-hour access, and annual wellness appointments in order to provide exceptional, high-quality care. With more time for patients, health care providers are able to customize and improve quality of care for each patient. The nurse practitioner (NP) role has expanded into concierge medicine. NPs in concierge medicine are responsible for supplying services as a part of a concierge medicine team, including wellness visits, care coordination, house calls, and other physical exams as needed. Employment opportunities are typically with a medical practice. Scope of practice varies by state.

EDUCATION REQUIREMENTS

RN preparation is required. A Master of Science in Nursing with advanced practice certification as an NP is required. Certification is available through the American Association of Nurse Practitioners and American Nurses Credentialing Center.

CORE COMPETENCIES/SKILLS NEEDED

- Experience in primary care
- Expertise in history taking and physical assessment
- Superior problem solving and critical thinking skills
- Excellent communication and interpersonal skills
- Excellent customer service skills
- Knowledge about the health care system and resources for patients
- Ability to work independently and as part of a team

RELATED WEBSITES AND PROFESSIONAL ORGANIZATIONS

- American Association of Colleges of Nursing (www.aacn.nche.edu)
- American Nurses Credentialing Center (www.nursecredentialing.org)

61 CONSULTANT

BASIC DESCRIPTION
A consultant is one who gives advice or provides specialized services on an hourly or contractual basis; nurse consultants can provide advice and/or services in a wide range of areas, such as research development, clinical areas of expertise (diabetes, cardiovascular disease), curriculum development, staffing of health care institutions, and so forth. A consultant might work or practice in virtually any and all aspects of the health care industry, including private practice. Health care in general, and nursing in particular, provides a wide range of opportunities for consultants. Services can be provided as part of a group effort or by an individual with a specific area of expertise.

EDUCATIONAL REQUIREMENTS
RN preparation is required; often additional education is required in the consultant's area of expertise. For example, research consultants would have PhD degrees and clinical consultants would have graduate degrees in their clinical area of specialization.

CORE COMPETENCIES/SKILLS NEEDED
- Independent functioning and team skills, with a clear focus on results that are contracted for by the client
- Entrepreneurial skills
- Communication skills
- Organizational skills
- Writing ability
- Leadership skills
- Project management skills

RELATED WEBSITE AND PROFESSIONAL ORGANIZATION
- National Nurses in Business Association (www.nnba.net)

CONTINENCE NURSE **62**

BASIC DESCRIPTION
The continence nurse—a specialty role—is responsible for assessing, planning, intervening, and evaluating care of patients who have urinary and/or fecal incontinence.

EDUCATIONAL REQUIREMENTS
An RN preparation and a minimum of a Bachelor of Science in Nursing are required. Certification as certified continence nurse is available from the Wound, Ostomy, and Continence Certification Board.

CORE COMPETENCIES/SKILLS NEEDED
- Strong assessment and verbal and written communication skills
- Knowledge of anatomy, physiology, and pathophysiology of the genitourinary and gastrointestinal systems
- Strong computer skills and some knowledge in data collection and interpretation
- Knowledge to involve in establishing care protocols and processes of care that relate to the care of patients with continence issues

RELATED WEBSITE AND PROFESSIONAL ORGANIZATION
- Wound, Ostomy, and Continence Nursing Certification Board (www.wocncb.org)

63 CONTINUING EDUCATION DIRECTOR

BASIC DESCRIPTION

A continuing education director is a leader who works with departmental directors to ensure educational goals are met. The director delegates tasks and initiatives to educators to ensure that nurses gain the knowledge they need to develop professionally and improve their practice. The director is responsible for the coordination of educational initiatives and their dissemination to the appropriate departments in a timely fashion. Employment is typically found in a hospital or health care system. The director of education may also play a role in development or revision of institutional policies and procedures.

EDUCATION REQUIREMENTS

RN preparation is required. A bachelor's degree in nursing and a master's degree in nursing or education are also necessary. Previous experience in education is highly desirable. Certification is also available.

CORE COMPETENCIES/SKILLS NEEDED

- High motivation
- Organizational skills
- Ability to collaborate and delegate
- Computer and technological skills
- Knowledge of learning theories and principles
- Ability to teach
- Excellent communication and leadership skills
- Ability to apply concepts to practice

RELATED WEBSITE AND PROFESSIONAL ORGANIZATION

- National League for Nursing (www.nln.org)

CORONARY CARE NURSE

BASIC DESCRIPTION
Coronary care nurses specialize in the care of patients who have acute and chronic coronary conditions requiring close assessment and monitoring. They also provide essential care in the patient's cardiac rehabilitation program. They need to be familiar with electrocardiogram rhythms, emergency cardiac care, and cardiovascular medications.

EDUCATIONAL REQUIREMENTS
RN preparation is required; a Bachelor of Science in Nursing is required in most positions. Basic life support and advanced cardiac life support certifications are also required; certification in cardiac vascular nursing is offered by the American Nurses Credentialing Center and the American Association of Critical-Care Nurses.

CORE COMPETENCIES/SKILLS NEEDED
- Ability to work in a fast-paced environment that requires quick decision making
- Excellent communication, analytical, and assessment skills
- Strong background knowledge of cardiovascular pathophysiology and pharmacology
- Strong computer skills for electronic health record documentation
- Strong leadership and delegation skills

RELATED WEBSITES AND PROFESSIONAL ORGANIZATIONS
- American Association of Cardiovascular and Pulmonary Rehabilitation (www.aacvpr.org)
- American Association of Critical-Care Nurses (www.aacn.org)
- American Nurses Credentialing Center (www.nursecredentialing.org/NurseSpecialties/CardiacVascular.aspx)
- Society for Vascular Nursing (www.svnnet.org)

65 CORRECTIONAL FACILITY NURSE

BASIC DESCRIPTION
The nurse who works in a correctional facility provides health care for all inmates. This includes case management, responding to episodes of acute illness, emergency call management, psychiatric evaluations, and assessment of new inmates. The patients are those with health problems related to chronic illness, AIDS, substance abuse, renal failure/dialysis, respiratory diseases, and terminal cancer.

EDUCATIONAL REQUIREMENTS
RN preparation is required. Positions are entry level, and orientation and assignment to a preceptor is required in most correctional facilities.

CORE COMPETENCIES/SKILLS NEEDED
The nurse who works in a correctional facility needs strong basic nursing skills, including:

- Ability to function independently
- Ability to respond to emergency situations
- Knowledge of mental health issues
- Health promotion and disease prevention skills
- Strong assessment skills

RELATED WEBSITE AND PROFESSIONAL ORGANIZATION
- Official Home of Corrections (www.corrections.com)

CRITICAL CARE NURSE 66

BASIC DESCRIPTION

Critical care nurses care for patients who are critically ill. They have a great deal of one-on-one contact with the patients and are often the main source of information for the family members. They are responsible for constantly monitoring the patient's condition, as well as recognizing any subtle changes. These nurses use a great amount of technology within their practice, and function as integral members of the multidisciplinary health care team. Critical care nurses must possess the ability to collaborate with other members of the health care team such as physicians, case managers, therapists, and, especially, other nurses. They are responsible for all care given to the patient, from medication administration to tracheotomy and other ventilator care, as well as constant monitoring of the patient for any alterations in status. Responsibilities include monitoring, assessment, vital sign monitoring, ventilatory management, medication administration, intravenous insertion and infusion, central line care, Swan–Ganz catheters, and maintenance of a running record of the patient's status. They must be prepared at all times to perform cardiopulmonary resuscitation and other life-saving techniques.

EDUCATIONAL REQUIREMENTS

RN preparation and advanced cardiac life support certification are required. A Bachelor of Science in Nursing and critical care nurse certification are preferred, and may be required depending on the institution. Most institutions require at least 1 to 2 years of medical–surgical experience, although some hospitals are offering extended preceptorships to selected new graduates. Previous critical care experience is desired. In addition to prior experience, many institutions require nurses to pass a critical care course, usually offered in the hospital, and to complete 4 to 6 weeks of orientation to the unit. Certification in critical care or cardiac medicine is available from the American Association of Critical Care Nursing Certification Corporation.

CORE COMPETENCIES/SKILLS NEEDED

- Excellent assessment skills, ability to detect very subtle changes in a patient's condition
- Strong organizational skills, ability to prioritize
- Communication skills and patient and family education skills
- Strong knowledge of anatomy and physiology, medications and their actions, interactions, side effects, and calculations

- Maturity and ability to handle end-of-life issues, such as when to cease life-prolonging interventions or organ donation decisions
- Affinity for technology

RELATED WEBSITE AND PROFESSIONAL ORGANIZATION
- American Association of Critical-Care Nurses (www.aacn.org)

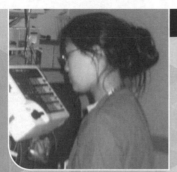

 PROFILE: **MAY LING LUC**
Critical Care Nurse

1. **What is your educational background in nursing (and other areas) and what formal credentials do you hold?**

I have a bachelor's degree in nursing and am a certified critical care nurse.

2. **How did you first become interested in your current career?**

The career found me. I originally majored in physical therapy in college; however, I lost interest in it and became exploratory for a semester until my advisor told me to try out nursing. She called the assistant dean of the school of nursing; I had a meeting with her; she looked at my credentials and said that I should transfer to the school of nursing. I did, and that summer I found out that I was going to be a nursing student. It was one of the best things that ever happened to me. I love doing what I do.

3. **What are the most rewarding aspects of your career?**

When patients are truly appreciative of what I do for them.

4. **What advice would you give to someone contemplating the same career path in nursing?**

Observe first; if you have a close friend who is a nurse, get his or her perspective on it. Also go for either your bachelor's or master's degree in nursing.

67 CRITICAL CARE TRANSPORT NURSE

BASIC DESCRIPTION
The critical care transport nurse (CCTN) provides essential services in ensuring the safe on-ground transfer of acutely ill patients from one health care facility to another. The CCTN assesses, monitors, intervenes, and stabilizes critically ill patients during transport.

EDUCATIONAL REQUIREMENTS
RN preparation and at least 2 years of critical care or emergency department experience are required; current basic life support, advanced cardiac life support, and pediatric advanced life support (PALS) certifications are required. Certification as a certified transport registered nurse is available from the Emergency Nurses Association and the Board of Certification for Emergency Nursing.

CORE COMPETENCIES/SKILLS NEEDED
- Ability to work in a high-stress environment
- Ability to lift or move objects over 80 pounds
- Excellent communication and assessment skills
- Strong computer skills and ability to use electronic health record/documentation effectively
- Strong clinical, critical thinking, and decision-making skills

RELATED WEBSITES AND PROFESSIONAL ORGANIZATIONS
- Air & Surface Transport Nurses Association (www.astna.org)
- Board of Certification for Emergency Nursing (www.bcencertifications.org)
- Emergency Nurses Association (www.ena.org)

CRUISE SHIP/RESORT NURSE

68

BASIC DESCRIPTION

Cruise ship/resort nurses work on ships or at resorts to provide emergency and general care to passengers and vacationers, should it be required. These nurses also serve as part of the occupational health team for crew members who live on the ship for 6 to 8 months at a time, or for the staff at resorts. Responsibilities include providing patient care in the health center and dealing with on-site emergencies. This work offers flexibility. Assignments are 3- to 6-month contract positions, living and working with the same people, and meeting people from around the world.

Responsibilities include:

- Providing patient care both on a day-to-day basis and in emergency situations
- Maintaining rapport with guests, physicians, and other crew members
- Communicating to arrange for workers or guests to receive medical attention
- Providing discharge instructions for each patient
- Preparing and maintaining medical records and billing for all patients
- Complying with resort and maritime rules, regulations, and procedures

EDUCATIONAL REQUIREMENTS

RN preparation with a minimum of 2 years of recent hospital experience is required. Experience with cardiac care, trauma, and internal medicine is desirable.

CORE COMPETENCIES/SKILLS NEEDED

- Excellent interpersonal skills; must enjoy traveling and must be flexible
- Excellent communication skills
- Strong health assessment skills
- A valid passport
- Ability to advise patients with colds, headaches, or other minor illnesses

RELATED WEBSITE AND PROFESSIONAL ORGANIZATION

- Cruise Line Employment (www.cruiselinejob.com/medical.htm)

69

DEAN OF HEALTH SCIENCES

BASIC DESCRIPTION
A dean is a head of a faculty or department in a college or university. A dean has a range of responsibilities that ultimately uphold the mission of the institution. Duties include maintaining optimal administrative and academic operations of the school, managing budgets and finance, providing leadership for strategic planning, being responsible for faculty, upholding academic standards and policies, preparing for accreditation, and leading the school toward constant growth and improvement.

EDUCATIONAL REQUIREMENTS
A doctorate degree in a health care–related field is required, with relevant academic leadership experience.

CORE COMPETENCIES/SKILLS NEEDED
- Academic integrity
- Experience in academic and administrative leadership
- Strong leadership and administrative skills
- Grant-writing and/or research-funding skills
- Ability to collaborate with a large number of people
- Excellent communication and interpersonal skills
- High motivation and commitment to excellence
- Familiarity with accrediting processes

RELATED WEBSITES AND PROFESSIONAL ORGANIZATIONS
- American Association of Colleges of Nursing (www.aacn.nche.edu)
- National League for Nursing (www.nln.org)

DEAN OF NURSING

BASIC DESCRIPTION
The dean of nursing is an administrative position in a school or college of nursing. Aside from providing academic and educational leadership to the faculty, students, and alumnae/i, the dean of nursing supervises faculty-related procedures that relate to instructional, research, and service programs; oversees the budgetary needs; and conducts evaluations of associate and assistant deans and chairs of the departments/colleges of the school.

EDUCATIONAL REQUIREMENTS
A master's degree or higher is required.

CORE COMPETENCIES/SKILLS NEEDED
- Strong administrative, interpersonal, and communication skills
- Strong background in organizational leadership and management, fiscal and budgetary affairs, and nursing research and education
- Knowledge of nursing curriculum and university/college policies
- Strong background in human resources–related matters

RELATED WEBSITES AND PROFESSIONAL ORGANIZATIONS
- American Association of Colleges of Nursing (www.aacn.nche.edu/ContactUs/index.htm)
- National League for Nursing (www.nln.org)

DERMATOLOGY NURSE

BASIC DESCRIPTION
This multifaceted job encompasses the full spectrum of patient care of those who have dermatological conditions. Dermatology nurses work in clinics, hospitals, and other health care settings. The job responsibilities include skin cancer screening, assistance in treatment, administrative work, and patient teaching.

EDUCATIONAL REQUIREMENTS
RN preparation is highly preferred; an initial 3-year certification is available from the Dermatology Nursing Certification Board, a member of the American Board of Nursing Specialties.

CORE COMPETENCIES/SKILLS NEEDED
- Excellent organizational and communication skills
- Knowledge of the physiology and pathophysiology in dermatology, and their treatment
- Continuing education credits for recertification

RELATED WEBSITES AND PROFESSIONAL ORGANIZATIONS
- American Board of Nursing Specialties (www.nursingcertification.org)
- Dermatology Nurses' Association (www.dnanurse.org)

DERMATOLOGY NURSE PRACTITIONER

72

BASIC DESCRIPTION
The dermatology nurse practitioner—an advanced practice role—is responsible for assessing, diagnosing, and treating common dermatological disorders, such as psoriasis, dermatitis, or eczema, and dermatological infections, such as those caused by viruses, fungi, or bacteria.

EDUCATIONAL REQUIREMENTS
A master's degree and a nurse practitioner certification are required; for certification as a dermatology certified nurse practitioner, a minimum of 3,000 hours of practice in dermatology is also required.

CORE COMPETENCIES/SKILLS NEEDED
- Excellent assessment skills
- Advanced knowledge of the physiology and pathophysiology in dermatology and their treatment
- Ability to work with collaborating dermatologist

RELATED WEBSITES AND PROFESSIONAL ORGANIZATIONS
- National Academy of Dermatology Nurse Practitioners (nadnp.enpnetwork.com)
- Nurse Practitioner Society of Dermatology Nurses' Association (www.dnanurse.org)

73 DEVELOPMENTAL DISABILITIES NURSE PRACTITIONER

BASIC DESCRIPTION
Developmental disabilities nurse practitioners are clinical experts in providing primary care to those who have cognitive and physical disabilities, such as mental retardation, autism, and Asperger's syndrome. Developmental disabilities nurse practitioners are also strong advocates in fostering improved knowledge about the care of patients who have developmental disabilities. They are employed in various settings, such as hospitals, schools, and primary care centers.

EDUCATIONAL REQUIREMENTS
RN preparation, nurse practitioner certification, and basic life support certification are required; certification as a developmental disabilities nurse is required in most positions.

CORE COMPETENCIES/SKILLS NEEDED
- Excellent communication and assessment skills
- Strong advocate for and commitment to the issues that relate to the care of patients who have developmental disabilities
- Strong computer and documentation skills
- Sensitivity to the unique needs of patients with developmental/learning disabilities and their families

RELATED WEBSITE AND PROFESSIONAL ORGANIZATION
- Developmental Disabilities Nurses Association (www.ddna.org)

DIABETES EDUCATOR

BASIC DESCRIPTION
The diabetes educator works with patients who have diabetes to teach them about the disease and how to live a healthy life with this very common health problem. Most diabetes educators work in clinics or physician offices and manage the care of clients with this disease. The diabetes nurse educator establishes long-term commitments and knows patients very well. Responsibilities include instruction on foot and skin care, and appropriate diet; monitoring of blood glucose; and administration of insulin. The diabetes educator must have extensive knowledge of diabetes and its management, and must keep up with the newest techniques and interventions available.

EDUCATIONAL REQUIREMENTS
The care of patients with diabetes is very complex and requires a minimum of a Bachelor of Science in Nursing and special certification as a diabetes educator. Increasingly, a Master of Science in Nursing is required. Certification is available from the National Certification Board for Diabetes Educators.

CORE COMPETENCIES/SKILLS NEEDED
- Extensive expertise and knowledge about the care of patients with diabetes, patient education skills, and interpersonal skills

RELATED WEBSITES AND NURSING ORGANIZATIONS
- American Association of Diabetes Educators (www.diabeteseducator.org)
- National Certification Board for Diabetes Educators (www.ncbde.org)

75 DIALYSIS NURSE

BASIC DESCRIPTION
A dialysis nurse—a specialized role in nephrology nursing—specifically provides care to patients undergoing dialysis or peritoneal dialysis. Dialysis is a life-saving and/or life-sustaining procedure performed in patients who have kidney failure.

EDUCATIONAL REQUIREMENTS
RN preparation is required; a Bachelor of Science in Nursing is highly preferred and basic life support certification is required. Certification as either a nephrology or dialysis nurse is available from the Board of Nephrology Examiners Nursing and Technology or from the Nephrology Nursing Certification Commission.

CORE COMPETENCIES/SKILLS NEEDED
- Knowledge and familiarity of equipment used for hemodialysis and peritoneal dialysis
- Strong interpersonal communication, assessment, and analytical skills
- Sensitivity to patient needs and their families

RELATED WEBSITES AND PROFESSIONAL ORGANIZATIONS
- American Nephrology Association (www.annanurse.org)
- Board of Nephrology Examiners Nursing and Technology (www.bonent.org)
- Nephrology Nursing Certification Commission (www.nncc-exam.org)

DISASTER/BIOTERRORISM NURSE

76

BASIC DESCRIPTION

The disaster/bioterrorism nurse works in disaster areas that are the result of a bioterrorist attack, or in situations caused by natural disaster, war, or poverty. Red Cross nurses are often part of the network that provides assistance during times of disaster or conflict. The nature of the work will vary depending on the course of the disaster or conflict.

EDUCATIONAL REQUIREMENTS

RN preparation is required. Red Cross nurses must have special training and 20 hours of volunteer or paid service before being assigned to a disaster situation.

CORE COMPETENCIES/SKILLS NEEDED

- Emergency department or critical care experience
- Experience with local disaster action teams
- Management skills
- Ability to meet the needs of people in crisis and high-stress situations
- Knowledge of disaster preparedness and basic first aid

RELATED WEBSITES AND PROFESSIONAL ORGANIZATIONS

- American Nurses Association: Bioterrorism and Disaster Response (www.nursingworld.org/disasterpreparedness)
- American Red Cross (www.redcross.org)

DISCHARGE PLANNER

BASIC DESCRIPTION
Discharge planners help patients through the discharge process from a hospital, skilled nursing facility, or rehabilitation facility. Their job is to ensure that a discharged patient has a safe plan to go home or to another residence facility. This includes assessing the needs of a patient, coordinating necessary services or equipment, proper transportation, follow-up care, and patient education. They also need to ensure patients understand their plan of care after leaving the health care facility. Discharge planners may spend time educating patients about new medications, explaining their diagnoses, and making follow-up appointments. They can also meet with patients to learn their discharge goals and address their concerns before they go home.

EDUCATIONAL REQUIREMENTS
RN preparation is required. Relevant experience as a clinical nurse is also necessary.

CORE COMPETENCIES/SKILLS NEEDED
- Excellent coordination and organizational skills
- Ability to educate patients
- Ability to collaborate with other health care providers
- Strong communication and interpersonal skills
- Understanding of community resources
- Familiarity with insurance reimbursement guidelines
- Ability to advocate for patients and their rights

RELATED WEBSITES AND PROFESSIONAL ORGANIZATIONS
There are no related websites or organizations.

DOMESTIC VIOLENCE NURSE EXAMINER

BASIC DESCRIPTION

These specialists are trained not only to care for patients who are survivors of domestic violence but also to spot signs of abuse and to accurately document evidence that could be used in legal proceedings. They work in various health care settings, such as emergency departments, ambulatory settings, shelters, and in advocacy groups, that serve domestic violence victims. They could also be trained mental health counselors or sexual assault nurse examiners (SANE).

EDUCATIONAL REQUIREMENTS

RN preparation is required. A Bachelor of Science in Nursing is preferred. Certification as SANE is preferred in most job positions; SANE certification is offered by the Forensic Nursing Certification Board.

CORE COMPETENCIES/SKILLS NEEDED

- Advanced knowledge in forensics and preparation as mental health counselor
- Excellent verbal and written communication skills
- Ability to provide sensitive and culturally appropriate care to victims of abuse
- Knowledge of resources and agencies that provide care and assistance to domestic violence victims

RELATED WEBSITES AND PROFESSIONAL ORGANIZATIONS

- Forensic Nursing Certification Board (www.forensicnurses.org/?page=Certification)
- International Association of Forensic Nursing (www.iafn.org)
- Nursing Network on Violence Against Women International (www.nnvawi.org)

79 DOULA

BASIC DESCRIPTION
A doula is a woman who is specially trained to provide assistance to women during labor and delivery. She offers education, provides assistance in development and execution of birth plans, facilitates communication between the mother and the care team, offers emotional support and assistance with newborn care. Doulas can work specifically during the birthing process or during the postpartum period.

EDUCATIONAL REQUIREMENTS
Special training in childbirth and childbirth education are required to be a doula. Certification from the International Doula Institute or DONA International is available and encouraged.

CORE COMPETENCIES/SKILLS NEEDED
- Complete understanding of the process and physiology of birth
- High emotional intelligence
- Ability to nurture and comfort a woman during childbirth
- Excellent verbal communication skills and interpersonal skills
- Ability to support and educate a mother and family about the childbirth process and care of the newborn

RELATED WEBSITES AND PROFESSIONAL ORGANIZATIONS
- American Pregnancy Association (www.americanpregnancy.org)
- Childbirth and Postpartum Professional Association (www.cappa.net)
- DONA International (www.dona.org)
- International Doula Institute (www.internationaldoulainstitute.com)

EAR, NOSE, AND THROAT NURSE

BASIC DESCRIPTION

Nurses in this area of practice deal with patients who have ear, nose, and throat (ENT) conditions. They work in various health care settings and cater to all patient populations. They could work in outpatient ENT clinics that cater to minor ENT problems or in special units that cater to complex ENT cases, such as those with maxillofacial trauma or those undergoing head and neck surgeries and chemotherapy.

EDUCATIONAL REQUIREMENTS

RN preparation is required; specialty certification is offered by the National Certifying Board of Otorhinolaryngology and Head-Neck Nurses.

CORE COMPETENCIES/SKILLS NEEDED

- Knowledge of ENT pathophysiology and its management
- Excellent interpersonal skills and sensitivity to the needs of patients who may have body image issues
- Strong computer skills and knowledge of electronic health record
- Ability to work in a team

RELATED WEBSITE AND PROFESSIONAL ORGANIZATION

- Society of Otorhinolaryngology and Head-Neck Nurses (sohnnurse.com)

81

EAR, NOSE, AND THROAT NURSE PRACTITIONER

BASIC DESCRIPTION

Ear, nose, and throat (ENT) nurse practitioners diagnose, treat, and evaluate patients who have ENT disorders. Other primary responsibilities include ordering diagnostic tests, providing health promotion education, assisting the surgeon in ENT surgeries, and evaluating patient progress and discharging patients as appropriate.

EDUCATIONAL REQUIREMENTS

RN preparation and nurse practitioner certification are required.

CORE COMPETENCIES/SKILLS NEEDED

- Advanced knowledge related to ENT pathophysiology and disease diagnosis, and medical–surgical and pharmacological management of patients who have ENT conditions
- Excellent interpersonal and communication skills
- Ability to work in a team
- Sensitivity to the needs of patients and their families and knowledge of resources and referral networks available

RELATED WEBSITE AND PROFESSIONAL ORGANIZATION

- Society of Otorhinolaryngology and Head-Neck Nurses (www.sohnnurse.com)

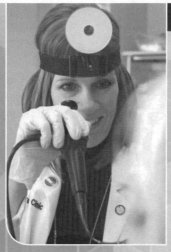

1. What is your educational background in nursing (and other areas) and what formal credentials do you hold?

I hold three degrees: Bachelor of Science in Nursing, Master of Science in Nursing, and Doctor of Nursing Practice. I am certified as an otorhinolaryngology and head-neck nurse, and I hold a certification from the American Nurses Credentialing Center as an adult nurse practitioner. I have more than 26 years of nursing experience.

2. How did you first become interested in your current career?

I first became interested in ENT nursing while working in the operating room (OR) and intensive care unit (ICU) at a major medical center. I began working with a prominent head and neck surgeon as a nurse clinician in his medical practice. The physician began to mentor and train me as he would have trained a medical resident or resident. I made rounds, cowrote orders, and assisted with the in-house patients. On the outpatient side, I was available in the office to triage calls, manage patients going through surgery, and perform small office procedures (removal of nasal packing, stitches, giving chemical peels, etc.). When I began my nurse practitioner training, the physician mentored me to another level. I began to do flexible nasal endoscopy, laryngoscopy, microscopic earwax removal, sinus/nasal debridement, and simple biopsies. My mentoring physician showed me the side of managing a patient practice. I was responsible for ordering supplies

Continued

and working with office assistants. The physician also encouraged me to join a professional nursing organization. I began to attend nursing meetings, began lecturing, and took on the role of coordinator of an ENT Nursing Review course. I became interested in leadership and was elected to the board of directors. I went on to become vice president of my professional nursing organization, the Society of Otorhinolaryngology and Head-Neck Nurses (SOHN).

3. What are the most rewarding aspects of your career?

I enjoy three things: Empowering my patients to live a healthy lifestyle, mentoring others about ENT nursing, and enjoying the flexibility that is offered by my current nursing position. I am able to balance my professional and family life.

4. What advice would you give to someone contemplating the same career path in nursing?

I would tell others to follow their instincts. Nursing is not a "catchall" profession. I would not advise someone to go into nursing for the money or the stability of a job. Go into nursing to give something back. Nursing can allow you many opportunities. I have worked in the OR, the ICU, and a medical–surgical floor; as a liver–kidney procurement coordinator, a preceptor, adjunct faculty, and—best of all—an ENT nurse practitioner. I have a great professional career, which has been balanced with family life. Many times I have been asked why I did not become a doctor. I simply reply, "because I love being a nurse." I found what I was meant to do. I have never looked back. No regrets.

EDITOR, BOOK

BASIC DESCRIPTION
This is a nurse who edits books and/or monographs for publication in print or through electronic media. The work may be in any scientific/professional content area in nursing and health care or related areas. This edited material may be used in research, education, training, sales and marketing, and other media and communication forms. The editor can be the originator of the content idea for the book, or can be hired by others to do the editing work. This specialty combines editing and writing skills with nursing and health care knowledge. There are numerous opportunities for freelance work that can be done from home with flexible hours. Sometimes the work can be isolating and the data can be very technical, detail oriented, tedious, and voluminous; however, the work varies depending on the content being edited. Opportunities exist to work for nursing and medical marketing/communications companies, pharmaceutical companies, nursing, medical and general interest publishing houses, nursing and medical education companies, and professional organizations.

EDUCATIONAL REQUIREMENTS
RN preparation is required; a Bachelor of Science in Nursing, or higher, is often required; content expertise is expected.

CORE COMPETENCIES/SKILLS NEEDED
- Excellent writing skills
- Good command of the English language
- Attention to detail
- Strong organizational and analytical skills
- Ability to work alone
- Ability to meet deadlines
- Excellent computer skills
- Health care–related knowledge

RELATED WEBSITES AND PROFESSIONAL ORGANIZATIONS
- American Copy Editors Society (www.copydesk.org)
- American Medical Writers Association (www.amwa.org)
- Board of Editors in the Life Sciences (www.bels.org)
- International Academy of Nursing Editors (www.nursingeditors-inane.org)
- Nurse Author & Editor (naepub.com)

83

EDITOR, JOURNAL

BASIC DESCRIPTION

This is a nurse who edits journals or other periodical publications, published in print or through electronic media. The work may be in any scientific/professional content area in nursing and health care or related areas. This edited material may be used in research, education, training, sales and marketing, and other media and communication forms. The editor of the journal/periodical is usually selected and contracted by the publishing company or professional organization that owns the publication. The editor is most often selected for both content expertise and editing/publication experience. This specialty combines editing and writing skills with nursing and health care knowledge. There are numerous opportunities for freelance work that can be done from home with flexible hours. Sometimes the work can be isolating and the data can be very technical, detail oriented, tedious, and voluminous; however, the work varies depending on the content being edited. Opportunities exist to work for major publishing companies in the health sciences, nursing and medical marketing/communications companies, pharmaceutical companies, general interest publishing houses, nursing and medical education companies, and professional organizations.

EDUCATIONAL REQUIREMENTS

RN preparation is required. A Bachelor of Science in Nursing, or higher, is often required; content expertise is expected.

CORE COMPETENCIES/SKILLS NEEDED

- Excellent writing skills
- Good command of the English language
- Attention to detail
- Strong organizational and analytical skills
- Ability to work alone
- Ability to meet deadlines
- Excellent computer skills
- Health care–related knowledge
- Ability to work with others, for example, editorial board members, association board members

RELATED WEBSITES AND PROFESSIONAL ORGANIZATIONS

- American Copy Editors Society (www.copydesk.org)
- American Medical Writers Association (www.amwa.org)

- American Society of Healthcare Publication Editors (www.ashpe.org)
- Board of Editors in the Life Sciences (www.bels.org)
- Committee on Publication Ethics (publicationethics.org)
- Council of Science Editors (www.councilscienceeditors.org)
- International Academy of Nursing Editors (www.nursingeditors-inane.org)
- International Committee of Medical Journal Editors (http://www.icmje.org)
- Nurse Author & Editor (www.nurseauthoreditor.com)

84 EDUCATOR

BASIC DESCRIPTION
College and university faculty who teach and advise students on basic and graduate degree programs in nursing are nurse educators or academic nurses. Faculty may give lectures to several hundred students in large halls, lead small seminars, or supervise students in laboratories. They prepare lectures, exercises, and laboratory experiments; grade exams and papers; and advise and work with students individually. In universities, they also supervise graduate students' teaching and research. Faculty members are expected to keep up with developments in their field by reading current literature and participating in professional conferences. Faculty members consult with governmental, business, nonprofit, and community organizations. They also do their own research to expand knowledge in their field. They perform experiments; collect and analyze data; and publish their research results in professional journals, books, and electronic media. Most faculty members serve on academic or administrative committees that deal with the policies of their institution, departmental matters, academic issues, curricula, budgets, equipment purchases, and hiring. Some work with student and community organizations. Department chairpersons are faculty members who usually teach some courses but have heavier administrative responsibilities. Clinical faculty members provide clinical supervision of students.

EDUCATIONAL REQUIREMENTS
Requirements vary with level of position. College faculty and deans usually need a doctorate (PhD, EdD, DNSc, DNP). These individuals serve as the top administrative officer of the academic unit for full-time, tenure-track, or non–tenure track positions in 4-year colleges and universities. Instructors and clinical faculty most often have educational preparation at the master's degree level. Certification is available from the National League for Nursing.

CORE COMPETENCIES/SKILLS NEEDED
- Strong interpersonal and communication skills
- Motivational and mentoring skills
- Knowledge of teaching/learning and/or management principles and practices
- Ability to make sound decisions and to organize and coordinate work efficiently
- Time management skills; ability to work independently and manage a large number of diverse projects

- Research and publication skills, especially for faculty at professorial ranks in colleges and universities
- Ability to manage a flexible schedule—faculty usually teach 12 to 16 hours per week—and to attend faculty and committee meetings. Most faculty establish regular office hours for student consultations, usually 3 to 6 hours per week. Faculty devote time to course preparation, grading, research, graduate student supervision, and other activities.

RELATED WEBSITES AND PROFESSIONAL ORGANIZATIONS

- American Association of Colleges of Nursing (www.aacn.nche.edu)
- National League for Nursing (www.nln.org)

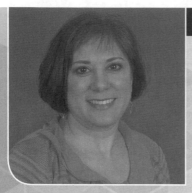

 PROFILE: CELESTE M. ALFES
Nurse Educator—University

1. What is your educational background in nursing (and other areas) and what formal credentials do you hold?

I hold three nursing degrees: Bachelor of Science in Nursing, Master of Science in Nursing (MSN) with a focus on nursing education, and Doctor of Nursing Practice (DNP) with a focus on nursing education.

2. How did you first become interested in your current career?

While in my undergraduate nursing program, I had the opportunity to work as a student nurse in various critical care units. In this position, I was fortunate to float to the intensive care unit (ICU), coronary care unit (CCU), medical ICU (MICU), and recovery room while working with various patients, nurses, and specialty physicians. Caring for cardiac patients was my favorite area and upon graduation, I worked in the CCU while completing my MSN. During my master's program, I also worked as a graduate teaching assistant in the skills lab at my school of nursing. I soon discovered how rewarding it was to teach young and highly motivated students how to be caring and effective nurses while delivering the highest level of care for their patients. During these 2 years as a graduate teaching assistant, it became clear I wanted to be a nurse educator.

3. What are the most rewarding aspects of your career?

As a nurse educator I am always surrounded by young professionals eager to learn, motivated to become nurses, committed to excellent patient care, and devoted to quality and safety. It is extremely rewarding to see young minds develop and individuals grow and mature into nursing professionals

Continued

you would want caring for you and your family members. Being a nurse educator provides the opportunity to be a role model, to shape the future of our nursing profession, and to challenge yourself and your students to stay current in an ever-changing health care system. As a nurse educator, I am also grateful that my position allows for a healthy work–life balance while I remain actively involved in the nursing profession.

4. What advice would you give to someone contemplating the same career path in nursing?

To become an effective nurse educator, I recommend working in a hospital on a unit or floor of your choice for 2 to 3 years, followed by enrolling in an MSN program to become an advanced practice nurse or nurse educator. I also advise working part time or on an as-needed basis as a staff nurse, becoming a graduate teaching assistant, and taking a course or two in nursing education. Be sure to take advantage of teaching opportunities in the hospital as a preceptor or mentor to see if you really do enjoy working with students or new nurses. Once you have completed your MSN and feel becoming a nurse educator is desirable, I would advise pursuing your DNP with a focus in nursing education. As a nurse educator of 23 years, I highly recommend exploring the dynamic and multifaceted opportunities nursing education provides.

85 ELECTROPHYSIOLOGY NURSE

BASIC DESCRIPTION
An electrophysiology nurse—a specialty in cardiology nursing—assists and educates patients undergoing an electrophysiology study procedure of the heart. An electrophysiology study of the heart involves a nonsurgical procedure to obtain information about the heart's electrical activity. The electrophysiology nurse also works with patients who have pacemakers or defibrillators.

EDUCATIONAL REQUIREMENTS
RN preparation and basic life support and advanced cardiac life support certifications are required. Certification is available from the American Nurses Credentialing Center as a cardiac–vascular nurse and from the American Association of Critical-Care Nurses as a critical care nurse.

CORE COMPETENCIES/SKILLS NEEDED
- Minimum acute care experience preferably in emergency nursing or critical care
- Strong knowledge in cardiology
- Excellent assessment and critical thinking skills

RELATED WEBSITES AND PROFESSIONAL ORGANIZATIONS
- American Association of Critical-Care Nurses (www.aacn.org)
- American Nurses Credentialing Center (www.nursecredentialing.org/NurseSpecialties/CardiacVascular.aspx)
- Preventive Cardiovascular Nurses Association (www.pcna.net)

EMERGENCY DEPARTMENT NURSE

86

BASIC DESCRIPTION

Emergency department (ED) nurses specialize in trauma and critical care, working in environments that are specially equipped to manage emergency care in life-threatening circumstances. ED nurses are often on the front line of health care, as many persons use the ED as their primary source of care.

EDUCATIONAL REQUIREMENTS

RN preparation with 1 to 3 years of acute care experience is required. Although not required by all EDs, ED nurses are usually trained in advanced cardiac life support and pediatric advanced life support. Certification is available from the Board of Certification for Emergency Nursing.

CORE COMPETENCIES/SKILLS NEEDED

- Organization skills
- Ability to triage patients
- Mental ability to deal with death and dying
- Ability to take medical histories and make accurate assessments quickly
- Ability to manage mass casualty situations
- Technical proficiency with health care equipment
- Ability to function in high-stress situations

RELATED WEBSITES AND PROFESSIONAL ORGANIZATIONS

- Emergency Nurses Association (www.ena.org)
- *Journal of Emergency Nursing* (www.jenonline.org)

87 EMERGENCY DEPARTMENT NURSE PRACTITIONER

BASIC DESCRIPTION
The emergency department (ED) nurse practitioner—an advanced practice role—delivers primary care in the ED. He or she could treat common urgent and nonemergency medical conditions in collaboration with the ED attending physician.

EDUCATIONAL REQUIREMENTS
RN preparation, nurse practitioner (NP) certification, and a Master of Science in Nursing are required. Previous experience in ER or critical care nursing is often required for the position. Certification as an acute care NP is offered by the American Nurses Credentialing Center and by the American Association of Critical-Care Nurses.

CORE COMPETENCIES/SKILLS NEEDED
- Excellent analytical and communication skills
- Advanced training and education in the care of critically ill patients
- Ability to work under pressure and make quick, important clinical decisions
- Excellent management and organizational skills and ability to work with members of the health care team
- Strong computer skills, especially in the use of electronic health record/documentation

RELATED WEBSITES AND PROFESSIONAL ORGANIZATIONS
- American Association of Critical-Care Nurses (www.aacn.org)
- American College of Nurse Practitioners (www.acnp.org)
- American Nurses Credentialing Center (www.nursecredentialing.org)

PROFILE: THERESA M. CAMPO
Emergency Nurse Practitioner

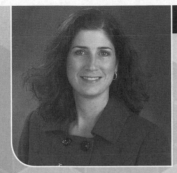

1. What is your educational background in nursing (and other areas) and what formal credentials do you hold?

After graduating from high school, I went the traditional route of becoming a nurse by obtaining a Diploma in Nursing. I then obtained a Bachelor of Science in Nursing (BSN), Master of Science in Nursing (MSN), and Doctor of Nursing Practice (DNP) degrees.

I am board certified as a family nurse practitioner (FNP) by the American Academy of Nurse Practitioners Certification Program and I am the first New Jersey advanced practice nurse to be board certified as an emergency nurse practitioner.

2. How did you first become interested in your current career?

I have always wanted to be a nurse since I was a young girl. I can't tell you why, but I can tell you it was what I strived for. I even dressed up as a nurse in kindergarten for "What do you want to be when you grow up?" day. In my early teenage years, I began to volunteer at my local hospital as a candy striper. I simply loved it! Right after my 16th birthday, I began to volunteer for my local ambulance service, and the next year I completed the requirements as a certified emergency medical technician (EMT). I worked summers as a medic on the Ocean City Beach Patrol and continued both of these fun-filled positions while attending nursing school at Ann May School of Nursing.

Once I graduated from nursing school, I worked on a medical–surgical unit and critical care unit before finally going to the emergency department, my life's dream! I was overwhelmed but loved the challenge. I was able to care for patients at their greatest hour of need and make a difference. I could also give comfort to family members and friends of patients and feel that I

Continued

made a difference on many levels. I loved the emergency department but I felt it was time to complete my BSN and see what the world had to offer.

One of my closest friends was considering going back to school for her BSN, so we decided to do it together. While pursuing my BSN degree, I was influenced by my friend's mother, who was a FNP. She was so intelligent and feisty and stood up for her patients, herself, and her NP position. I wanted to be just like her! Teresa Byrd and I both applied and were accepted to Widener University and about 3 years later completed our MSN in the FNP program. It was great. My mentor, Jan Town—an FNP whom I looked up to—was my preceptor during my MSN and I learned so much from her. I accepted a position in a cardiology practice and learned so much more than I could have ever imagined, yet it just didn't seem right to me. I was offered a position in the emergency department and accepted it.

Wow, was I fish out of water! I thought that since I worked in the emergency department as a nurse I could easily work there as an NP. Well, that was not the case. I had to interpret my own diagnostic tests (e.g., x-rays, lab values, EKG) and perform procedures that I had earlier assisted with as a nurse. I was lucky enough to have supportive physicians and NPs who taught me every day how to get better at these skills.

3. What are the most rewarding aspects of your career?

The most rewarding aspects are my education, my colleagues, and most of all my patients. I have been given so many opportunities that would not have been possible without my education and practice. I have been in emergency medicine for almost 30 years, ranging from prehospital to fast track, emergency, and trauma. The things that stick out most for me are becoming a nurse and an NP. Both afforded me the opportunity to care for patients and their families in ways that are rewarding. I have learned more from caring for patients than from any book or journal. I always say, "Patients don't read the textbooks." You need to be aware that patients are individuals with very different needs. My grandmother always said the best school was the school of hard knocks. Experience is priceless and the best education you can get.

Having mentors who are nonjudgemental and support you and your abilities is so important. They see things in you that you don't see and are able to bring them out. That is a true gift. Stepping out of your comfort zone

Continued

PROFILE: THERESA M. CAMPO
Continued

is not easy, but once you do, a whole new world opens up. You have to trust in yourself, and helping to instill that self-confidence is what my mentors have done for me. I would not be able to list myself as an author, editor, entrepreneur, academic, and clinician without their guidance and support. The ability to take these lessons learned and give back to other nurses is wonderful. The pride I feel when I see my colleagues achieve their goals is amazing!

Recently, I have had the honor of helping to build a new organization for emergency nurse practitioners, the American Academy of Emergency Nurse Practitioners. This organization, and the people who developed and work with it every day, truly live the mission and vision. The organization supports emergency nurse practitioners partnering through collaborative practice with our nursing, physician, physician assistant, and other health professional colleagues to provide safe, high-quality patient care. It has affected my life and career in ways I could not have imagined.

Also, during my doctoral education, I developed many strong connections. I learned the power of networking, and opportunities that came from those experiences are priceless.

4. What advice would you give to someone contemplating the same career path in nursing?

My first recommendation would be to sit down, really think about what you want to do, and ask yourself if nursing, in any aspect, is right for you. Nursing is a way of life and living. It reaches every part of your body and soul. Yet it brings you rewards nothing else on this earth can give you. If it doesn't, then you may need to reevaluate your goals and ideals. If nursing is for you, then I say full speed ahead! Find a mentor to help you along your journey of education and practice; a mentor who sees in you what you do not; someone who can bring out your inner strengths when you feel you don't have any. Study hard, work hard, and pamper your inner you.

The next thing I recommend is to set your sights high, even in areas where you don't think you can achieve your goals—and find a way. Nurture your dreams and goals and reevaluate them frequently. Be open to ideas and opportunities because you never know where they may lead you. Look around for signs to guide you on your path; listen to your inner voice and trust it. I guarantee you it will never let you down if you listen to it.

In my opinion, nursing is a gift and an honor for which I am truly grateful.

88 EMERGING DISEASES MANAGER

BASIC DESCRIPTION

An emerging diseases manager is a leader who manages a group of health care specialists and is responsible for developing and operationalizing institutional plans relating to emerging diseases. This person manages the team that will develop projects and response plans, gather knowledge, and initiate plans to combat or prevent emerging diseases and to present emergency planning. This person also works closely with the Centers for Disease Control and Prevention and other government agencies to collect and share data and information.

EDUCATIONAL REQUIREMENTS

RN preparation is required. A bachelor's degree in nursing is required. A master's degree in nursing or a health care–related field is desirable.

CORE COMPETENCIES/SKILLS NEEDED

- Excellent oral and written communication skills
- Knowledge of emergency management and protocols
- Ability to collect and interpret data
- Ability to develop strong relationships with governmental agencies
- Strong leadership and interpersonal skills
- Knowledge of communicable and emerging diseases and emergency management planning
- Ability to work independently and as a member of a team

RELATED WEBSITE AND PROFESSIONAL ORGANIZATION

- Centers for Disease Control and Prevention (www.cdc.gov)

ENDOCRINOLOGY NURSE

BASIC DESCRIPTION

An endocrinology nurse is someone who specializes in the care of patients who have endocrine disorders, such as diabetes mellitus and Cushing's disease. These nurses work across age groups and are employed in various health care settings, such as inpatient hospital units or departments or ambulatory centers. Some endocrinology nurses are also specialists, such as a pediatric endocrinology nurse.

EDUCATIONAL REQUIREMENTS

RN preparation is required. A Bachelor of Science in Nursing is highly preferred; basic life support certification is required.

CORE COMPETENCIES/SKILLS NEEDED

- Strong knowledge of the endocrine and hormonal systems
- Excellent interpersonal communication, assessment, and analytical skills
- Sensitivity to the needs of patients and their families
- Strong computer skills, including the use of electronic health record documentation
- Ability to work in a team
- Strong organizational and leaderships skills, especially for those who have administrative duties commonly found in ambulatory endocrine centers

RELATED WEBSITES AND PROFESSIONAL ORGANIZATIONS

- American Diabetes Association (www.diabetes.org)
- Endocrine Nurses Society (www.endo-nurses.org)
- Pediatric Endocrinology Nursing Society (www.pens.org)
- Society for Endocrinology (www.endocrinology.org)

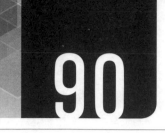

90 ENDOSCOPY NURSE

BASIC DESCRIPTION
Endoscopy nurses are responsible for providing nursing care for those patients, of all age groups, undergoing endoscopic procedures. They are employed in various settings, such as ambulatory centers or inpatient endoscopy units.

EDUCATIONAL REQUIREMENTS
RN preparation and current basic life support certification are required. Most facilities require at least 2 years of acute care experience. Most positions require certification in gastroenterology available from the American Board of Certification for Gastroenterology Nurses.

CORE COMPETENCIES/SKILLS NEEDED
- Ability to physically assist patients during endoscopic procedures that could include lifting, bending, pushing, and pulling
- Adequate manual dexterity
- Knowledge of basic electrocardiogram rhythms and dysrhythmia, and effects of sedation
- Ability to effectively communicate with patients and with members of the interprofessional team
- Strong computer and documentation skills

RELATED WEBSITE AND PROFESSIONAL ORGANIZATION
- American Board of Certification for Gastroenterology Nurses (www.abcgn .org)

ENDOSCOPY NURSE PRACTITIONER

BASIC DESCRIPTION
The endoscopy nurse practitioner provides primary care to those patients undergoing endoscopic procedures. Aside from performing or assisting in endoscopy, he or she also provides postprocedure follow-up and patient education, and discharges patients once stable.

EDUCATIONAL REQUIREMENTS
RN preparation, nurse practitioner certification, and basic life support/advanced cardiac life support certification are required. Acute clinical experience as an RN is also required. Certification as a gastroenterology nurse and training in gastroenterology medicine are required in most job positions.

CORE COMPETENCIES/SKILLS NEEDED
- Excellent assessment and analytical skills
- Ability to sit or stand in the endoscopy suite for an extended period of time, and ability to physically assist patients with lifting, bending, pushing, or pulling
- Strong leadership and organizational skills
- Advanced knowledge related to the physiology, pathophysiology, and pharmacological management of the gastrointestinal system
- Ability to effectively communicate with patients and with members of the interprofessional team

RELATED WEBSITE AND PROFESSIONAL ORGANIZATION
- American Board of Certification for Gastroenterology Nurses (www.abcgn .org)

92

ENTREPRENEUR

BASIC DESCRIPTION

An entrepreneur is a person who starts his or her own business, assuming all risk and responsibility. Nurse entrepreneurs may work in any aspect of the health care or medical industry. Examples of settings include independent practice, corporations, and industry.

EDUCATIONAL REQUIREMENTS

RN preparation is required. A Bachelor of Science in Nursing and a Master of Science in Nursing are desired. A degree in business is helpful.

CORE COMPETENCIES/SKILLS NEEDED

- A desire to have own business or practice independently
- Excellent communication skills
- Ability to be independent, flexible, autonomous, and have creative freedom
- Self-motivation, ambition, determination, and self-confidence
- Willingness to take risks and make important decisions

RELATED WEBSITES AND PROFESSIONAL ORGANIZATIONS

- National Nurses in Business Association (nnbanow.com)
- U.S. Small Business Administration (www.sba.gov)

PROFILE: JEAN AERTKER
Nurse Entrepreneur

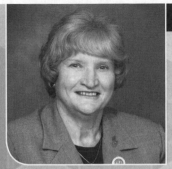

1. What is your educational background in nursing (and other areas) and what formal credentials do you hold?

I began my professional nursing career in 1973 with an Associate of Science in Nursing (ASN) and was one of the few commissioned into the United States Air Force (USAF) Nurse Corps with the ASN degree; I was commissioned in 1974. I completed the Baccalaureate of Science in Nursing (BSN) degree and then pursued a master's in nursing with a nurse practitioner focus. I completed a Doctor of Nursing Practice course in 2008. I am a board-certified nurse practitioner.

2. How did you first become interested in your current career?

While serving as an officer in the USAF Nurse Corps in 1974, I was introduced to the then-evolving role of the nurse practitioner. While the role seemed limited to pediatrics and women's health in the early years, nurse practitioners began to work more in the outpatient primary care clinics and family practice areas. The opportunity to promote health and wellness before illness or chronic disease states erupted seemed the best fit for my future nursing career and interest.

3. What are the most rewarding aspects of your career?

The reward of extensive education and leadership opportunities gave me the confidence to be a successful nurse entrepreneur and build my own practice by 1998. With this independence of ownership, I have a greater flexibility to be a mentor and consultant to new nurse practitioners and nursing colleagues in the profession. My role enables me to be more visible as an expert nurse in the community and in the workplace. It is a privilege to represent nursing through a business perspective.

Continued

PROFILE: JEAN AERTKER
Continued

4. What advice would you give to someone contemplating the same career path in nursing?

The educational ladder beginning with an ASN has value for those who plan to enter the world of work in nursing promptly, but it should not end there. I consider it the first rung on the ladder from which to build and develop the necessary skills and knowledge to care for patients in a very complex health care system. Nursing students today have many educational options, which can be very confusing. The program of choice must meet the needs of the student, family, and community, which includes the nursing profession. Nursing has long debated the appropriate degree for entry into professional nursing, but whatever route the student chooses, he or she must know there are many personal rewards in achieving the highest level of education in order to serve others and the profession.

93

BASIC DESCRIPTION
A nurse epidemiologist investigates trends in groups or aggregates and studies the occurrence of diseases and injuries. The information is gathered from census data, vital statistics, and reportable disease records. Nurse epidemiologists identify people or populations that are at high risk; monitor the progress of diseases; specify areas of health care need; determine priorities, size, and scope of programs; and evaluate their impact. They generally do not provide direct patient care, but serve as a resource and plan educational programs. They also publish results of studies and statistical analyses of morbidity and mortality. Examples of practice settings are the Centers for Disease Control and Prevention in Atlanta, Georgia; public health departments; and governmental agencies.

EDUCATIONAL REQUIREMENTS
A master's degree in public health or community health nursing is required. A PhD is preferred.

CORE COMPETENCIES/SKILLS NEEDED
- Mathematical and analytical ability
- Knowledge of both infectious and noninfectious diseases
- A desire to improve the health and well-being of populations
- Ability to identify populations at risk
- Knowledge of health policy
- Ability to plan programs and health services

RELATED WEBSITES AND PROFESSIONAL ORGANIZATIONS
- Association for Professionals in Infection Control and Epidemiology (www.apic.org)
- Centers for Disease Control and Prevention (www.cdc.gov)

94 ETHICIST

BASIC DESCRIPTION
A nurse ethicist is a person who knows about legal/moral/ethical issues and provides services for patients and families. The nurse ethicist may work with an ethics team to develop a detailed investigative plan to answer questions raised by an ethics violation allegation or resolve ethical dilemmas. Opportunities exist to work in hospitals, nursing homes, hospices, and outpatient settings.

EDUCATIONAL REQUIREMENTS
RN preparation and a Master of Science in Nursing or a graduate degree in bioethics or a related field are required.

CORE COMPETENCIES/SKILLS NEEDED
- Technical training and prior experience with investigations
- Excellent communication skills
- Ability to conduct and document investigations
- Ability to interview and/or review documents that may pertain to the allegations
- Knowledge of ethical and legal issues surrounding end-of-life care
- Knowledge of compliance-related concepts, policies, and procedures
- Ability to work well with others to draw conclusions based on allegations
- Expertise in pain management and issues of loss and grief

RELATED WEBSITES AND PROFESSIONAL ORGANIZATIONS
- Hospice Foundation of America (www.hospicefoundation.org)
- Johns Hopkins Berman Institute of Bioethics (www.bioethicsinstitute.org)
- Nursing World Ethics (www.nursingworld.org/ethics)

EVIDENCE-BASED PRACTICE DIRECTOR

95

BASIC DESCRIPTION
An evidence-based practice director is a nurse who is responsible for professional practice in a health care facility. This individual works collaboratively with a multidisciplinary team to ensure that best practice is being applied. Responsibilities include education, training, competency assessments, and management and oversight of nursing practice and patient safety.

EDUCATIONAL REQUIREMENTS
RN preparation and a master's degree in nursing are required. A doctoral degree is preferred. Relevant clinical and management experience is required.

CORE COMPETENCIES/SKILLS NEEDED
- Management and leadership skills
- Knowledge of Centers for Medicare & Medicaid Services (CMS) and The Joint Commission regulatory requirements
- Ability to be engaged and motivated
- Excellent communication skills
- Ability to teach and knowledge of various teaching methods
- Ability to work as an individual or as part of a team

RELATED WEBSITES AND PROFESSIONAL ORGANIZATIONS
- American Association of Colleges of Nursing (www.aacn.nche.edu)
- National Institute of Nursing Research (www.ninr.nih.gov)

96 FAMILY NURSE PRACTITIONER

BASIC DESCRIPTION
Family nurse practitioners (FNPs) are advanced practice nurses who specialize in providing health promotion and care to patients in primary care settings. FNPs provide primary screenings and focus on health promotion and disease prevention across the life span. They have many of the same duties as acute care practitioners, but typically do not work with patients who are critically ill. They perform physical examinations, order diagnostic tests, establish diagnoses, prescribe medications, and educate patients and family members regarding health and illness conditions and treatment plans. Examples of settings in which an FNP might practice are physicians' offices, health care clinics, private practice, hospitals, long-term care facilities, public health departments, and occupational health settings.

EDUCATIONAL REQUIREMENTS
A Master of Science in Nursing degree with advanced practice certification as an FNP is required. Programs are generally of 2 years' duration combining clinical and didactic work. Certification is available from the American Nurses Credentialing Center.

CORE COMPETENCIES/SKILLS NEEDED
- Ability to perform physical examinations
- Ability to assess accurately when doing screenings and diagnostic tests; knowledge of normal ranges and abnormal findings
- Strong communication skills
- Teaching ability and interest
- Ability to work with interdisciplinary teams as well as to function independently
- Knowledge of acute and chronic conditions
- Excellent judgment in knowing when to make a referral
- Ability to prescribe medications

RELATED WEBSITES AND PROFESSIONAL ORGANIZATIONS
- American Association of Nurse Practitioners (www.aanp.org)
- American Nurses Credentialing Center (www.nursecredentialing.org)

FAMILY PSYCHIATRIC–MENTAL HEALTH NURSE PRACTITIONER

BASIC DESCRIPTION

Family psychiatric–mental health nurse practitioners work with families to provide a full range of mental health care that includes assessing, diagnosing, and managing mental health issues. They may possess advanced training in psychotherapy, symptom management, and psychopharmacology. They treat various conditions that include bipolar disorders, schizophrenia, depression, and anxiety.

EDUCATIONAL REQUIREMENTS

RN preparation and nurse practitioner certification are required. Certification from the American Nurses Credentialing Center also is available. Experience as a mental health RN is preferred in most positions.

CORE COMPETENCIES/SKILLS NEEDED

- Advanced knowledge in mental health
- Sensitivity to patients and their families
- Excellent verbal and written communication skills
- Strong computer and documentation skills
- Ability to work as a member of a team

RELATED WEBSITES AND PROFESSIONAL ORGANIZATIONS

- American Nurses Credentialing Center (www.nursingcredentialing.org)
- American Psychiatric Nurses Association (www.apna.org)
- International Society of Psychiatric–Mental Health Nurses (www.ispn-psych.org)

98 FIRST ASSIST NURSE

BASIC DESCRIPTION
The registered nurse first assist (RNFA) works alongside the surgeon during the perioperative phase. The RNFA has undergone additional training to help surgeons in preoperative skin preparation, controlling surgical site bleeding, suturing, cutting, and cleansing surgical areas and applying dressings.

EDUCATIONAL REQUIREMENTS
RN preparation, Certified Nurse Operating Room certification, completion of postbasic nursing study that meets Association of periOperative Registered Nurses (AORN) standards for an RNFA education program, basic life support certification, and successful passing of the Certified Registered Nurse First Assistant certification examination are required for practice. Certification is also available from the Competency and Credentialing Institute.

CORE COMPETENCIES/SKILLS NEEDED
- Excellent communication skills
- Significant experience and knowledge in perioperative nursing
- Ability to work collaboratively with members of the perioperative team

RELATED WEBSITES AND PROFESSIONAL ORGANIZATIONS
- Association of periOperative Registered Nurses (www.aorn.org)
- Competency and Credentialing Institute (www.cc-institute.org)
- Registered Nurses First Assist Home (www.rnfa.org)

FLIGHT NURSE

99

BASIC DESCRIPTION
A flight nurse is a highly trained and experienced critical care RN. The flight nurse works with a flight crew most likely consisting of the flight nurse or paramedic, flight respiratory therapist or basic emergency medical technician (EMT-1), and a pilot to transport patients to, from, and between hospital facilities. Flight nurses work in intensive care units, emergency rooms, ambulance companies, and emergency transport facilities.

EDUCATIONAL REQUIREMENTS
RN preparation and a Bachelor of Science in Nursing are required. Strongly preferred are certification as a certified flight RN, certified emergency nurse, or certified critical care nurse, and as a prehospital provider. In addition, advanced cardiac life support and pediatric advanced life support, neonatal advanced life support, and completion of a trauma nurse core curriculum and of a flight nurse advanced trauma course are expected. This versatile practice usually requires a minimum of 2 to 3 years of critical care nursing experience. Rigorous ongoing continuing education is necessary to support the extensive unique knowledge and skills that are expected for flight nurses.

CORE COMPETENCIES/SKILLS NEEDED
- Experience with multisystem trauma, neonates, pediatrics, severe burns, acute medical care, high-risk obstetrics, and cardiac patients
- Ability to utilize endotracheal intubation and chemical paralytic agents; obtain central venous access via the femoral or subclavian route and intraosseous access; insert surgical airways; and perform pericardiocentesis or needle thoracostomy
- Responsibility of sharing knowledge about emergency care systems with other members of the health care team, patients, their significant others, and the community
- Involvement in research that directly relates to improved patient care in the air medical transport industry, and/or improves the professional standards of practice that promote the flight nurse as a professional
- Responsibility for direct patient care during transport that may include monitoring, medication administration, assessment, continued surveillance, IV infusion, ventilatory or airway management, charting, and communication with other health care providers

- Ability to provide rapid assessment, diagnosis, and treatment of critically injured or ill patients of all ages from the scene of an accident or from referring facilities

RELATED WEBSITES AND PROFESSIONAL ORGANIZATIONS

- Air & Surface Transport Nurses Association (www.astna.org)
- Dorothy Ebersbach Academic Center for Flight Nursing (www.flightnurse.case.edu)
- Nightingale International (www.NGI-MED.com)

PROFILE: CHRISTOPHER MANACCI

Acute Care Nurse Practitioner and
Flight Nurse Specialist

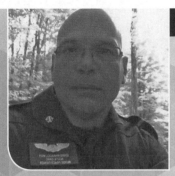

1. What is your educational background and preparation?

I have Bachelor of Science in Nursing, as well as Master of Science in Nursing and Doctor of Nursing Practice degrees. I am board certified as an acute care nurse practitioner from the Association of Critical-Care Nurses (AACN), board certified in flight nursing (CFRN), and certified as a trauma nurse specialist by the state of Illinois Department of Public Health.

2. How did you first become interested in your current career?

I first became interested in flight nursing (a new specialty at the time) while I was practicing in the intensive care unit (ICU) at a large community-based hospital. I enjoyed the complexity of the ICU patient population, but wanted to practice in an environment that required more acute intervention and stabilization. I trained as a trauma nurse specialist, then transitioned to the emergency department of an urban, level-one trauma center. After several years of practice, I missed the level of sophistication and detail the ICU patient population presented to my practice. Flight nursing combines the sophistication of an ICU with the urgency of an emergency department. It seemed like the "best of both worlds" as I was looking to increase my level of practice and capability. I continued my formal education to enhance my abilities to contribute to the body of knowledge in the specialty of flight nursing.

3. What are the most rewarding aspects of your career?

There is no question that I am granted the greatest privilege of any professional within or outside the health profession. On a daily basis I am given the privilege to care for the most critical of patients in their greatest time of need. My practice spans all age groups in every clinical subspecialty. I am able to be the human interface of the most technologically advanced

Continued

interventions, while encouraging physiological survival. Also, I serve as a link to individuals, families, and communities who may otherwise not benefit from access to specialty care centers. Since the inception of air medical services, nurses have always been the clinician of choice owing to their unique academic preparation in the physical, psychological, and social sciences, along with the clinical knowledge, critical thinking skills, and intervention capabilities inherent to our profession. Today, with the health care system under such immense scrutiny, I am proud to be a part of "what is right" about the health care system. I believe it was the French philosopher Voltaire who said, "Men who save lives partake in divinity, whereas saving a life is almost as noble as creating one." It is nurses who have the greatest opportunity to achieve this for those whose lives might otherwise end in tragedy.

On any given "typical" day, the only certainty is uncertainty. I report for duty at 7:00 a.m. and receive a report from the off-going flight nurse specialist including tasks such as reviewing pending missions, current and near-future weather conditions, evaluation of air worthiness of fellow crew members and aircraft, and accounting of narcotics stored. Then I prepare for and complete my routine duties of the shift, such as checking expiration dates and temperature range of stored blood used for missions. I am scheduled for 12- or 24-hour shifts. First I check the equipment and supplies aboard the S-76 aircraft (helicopter). This is essential as I do not have the luxury of calling CSR (central supply room) or pharmacy for missing items as the need may arise when I am caring for a patient on a freeway, in a cornfield, or at 1,500 feet while moving at 180 mph. We provide foundational nursing care, such as assessment, planning, intervention, and evaluation, as well as technically advanced procedures of airway management, central line placement, tube thoracostomy, and emergent surgical interventions. Preplanning for the unknown is the common denominator in flight nursing practice. There is no way to anticipate what type of mission awaits you, but a mission of some type is certain. On any given day you may care for an adult with a life-threatening medical condition or a young child critically injured in a car crash, or both in the same shift. You may be called for a high-risk obstetrical patient or a premature infant born with a congenital heart defect. Nonetheless, you will be called and need to be prepared for what awaits you.

Continued

4. What advice would you give to someone contemplating the same career path in nursing?

Every specialty in nursing provides you with unique opportunities, but flight nursing provides you with all of them. It is necessary to have a strong clinical background in critical care nursing and a strong understanding of pathophysiology, pharmacology, and clinical management of a variety of disease processes. It is essential that you enjoy caring for critically ill and injured patients in an unstructured environment. The best preparation is to be clinically proficient and trained and experienced in the concept of autonomous and collaborative practice. I believe it is helpful if you have completed research related to the care of individuals and have the ability to evaluate and implement current therapeutic interventions. The most important asset is the desire to make a difference and the passion to alter the outcome of those entrusted to your care.

Obtain as much formal education and clinical knowledge as early in your career as possible, do not jump from unit to unit; rather, understand the practice expectations in the process of caring for patients. This, coupled with clinical expertise and skill proficiencies, will provide you with the ability to be a strong candidate for a flight nursing position. More importantly, it will provide you with the tools to care for your patients in any setting.

100 FORENSIC NURSE

BASIC DESCRIPTION
Forensic nurses combine clinical nursing practice with knowledge of law enforcement. They provide care to victims and are involved in the investigation of sexual assault, elder and spousal abuse, and unexplained or accidental death. Forensic nursing is high stress because of the nature of the work, and it requires a broad understanding of social, environmental, and psychological influences on behavior. The environments in which forensic nurses work are varied. They work in such settings as correctional institutions, psychiatric facilities, acute care settings, coroner and medical examiners' offices, and for insurance companies.

EDUCATIONAL REQUIREMENTS
RN preparation and a Bachelor of Science in Nursing are required. Often, graduate preparation is required. Certification as a sexual assault nurse examiner may also be needed for some practice settings.

CORE COMPETENCIES/SKILLS NEEDED
- Ability to work in diverse conditions and deal with emotionally charged issues
- Ability to combine nursing knowledge with investigative and counseling skills
- Ability to collaborate with experts in other disciplines
- Ability to be an advocate for victims
- Skills to coordinate programs in collaboration with medical and law enforcement
- Ability to deal with death and dying

RELATED WEBSITE AND PROFESSIONAL ORGANIZATION
- International Association of Forensic Nurses (www.forensicnurses.org)

FOUNDATION EXECUTIVE

BASIC DESCRIPTION

A foundation executive is the administrative leader for a given organization. One may assume a variety of roles as a foundation executive, such as the chief executive officer (CEO), vice president, chief nursing officer, or director. A nurse can bring leadership expertise as a foundation executive with his or her unique health care experience to help advance the organization in accordance with the mission, vision, and values. The foundation executive most often serves as an ex-office member of the foundation board.

EDUCATIONAL REQUIREMENTS

Educational requirements vary based on the foundation's mission and goals. A bachelor's degree and a master's degree are usually required. A doctoral degree and related certifications are highly preferred.

CORE COMPETENCIES/SKILLS NEEDED

- Excellent communication skills
- Creativity and decisiveness
- Strong interpersonal and networking skills
- Willingness to take risks
- Knowledge of business and financial skills
- Experiential background relevant to foundation and position within the foundation
- Marketing skills
- Knowledge and experience in fundraising
- Excellent professional, leadership, and management skills
- Creativity and ability to solve problems
- Ability to be objective, resilient, and assertive
- Ability to work independently or collaborate and work well with a team

RELATED WEBSITES AND PROFESSIONAL ORGANIZATIONS

- American Nurses Foundation (www.anfonline.org)
- American Organization of Nurse Executives (www.aone.org/aone-foundation)
- Council for Advancement and Support of Education (www.case.org)
- Philanthropic organizations

102 FRAUD AND ABUSE INVESTIGATOR

BASIC DESCRIPTION

Fraud and abuse investigators examine health care fraud and abuse charges using such techniques as information technology and statistics to identify outlier practice behaviors. They are employed by government agencies or by independent consulting groups that perform services through contacts with government agencies. This allows investigators to recognize and look more closely at providers who are practicing in an unusual manner. Investigations are often aggressive and involve working with the FBI and U.S. attorneys to achieve justice. Cases are also reported to local medical and professional boards. The most common types of fraud and abuse are upcoding (e.g., a practitioner billing for a 60-minute office visit when it was only a 20-minute visit); unbundling, usually dealing with Current Procedural Terminology coding (e.g., a blood test being billed under a combined code, then one or more tests from that composite test being billed individually); charging for services not rendered; and performing unnecessary procedures or tests.

EDUCATIONAL REQUIREMENTS

RN preparation and an undergraduate degree are the baseline on which to add additional skills, certifications, and expertise. A graduate degree in business is desirable.

CORE COMPETENCIES/SKILLS NEEDED

- Computer literacy; understanding of information technology to deal with myriad databases
- A broad background in nursing with up-to-date clinical knowledge
- Experience and understanding of the health care system
- Study in law-related areas and in-depth understanding of managed care, risk management, and contracts
- Understanding of annual reports and budgets
- Understanding of statistics
- Appreciation of the cost of fraud

RELATED WEBSITE AND PROFESSIONAL ORGANIZATION

- New York State Bureau of Special Investigations
  Electronic Data Systems (www.health.ny.gov/prevention/nutrition/investigations)

GASTROENTEROLOGY NURSE

BASIC DESCRIPTION

Gastroenterology nursing is a specialty practice area in which nurses provide care to patients with known or suspected gastrointestinal problems and who are undergoing diagnostic or therapeutic treatment and/or procedures. This area of nursing has expanded because of increased technology and new screening procedures. Practice environments are usually available in endoscopy departments in hospitals, clinics, or physicians' offices, as well as in ambulatory outpatient endoscopy facilities.

EDUCATIONAL REQUIREMENTS

RN preparation is required. National certification in the specialty is available through the Certifying Board of Gastroenterology Nurses. This board sets the requirements for obtaining and maintaining certification. Certified registered nurses earn the credential "certified gastroenterology registered nurse." Generally, nurses have experience in medical–surgical nursing prior to electing to specialize.

CORE COMPETENCIES/SKILLS NEEDED

- Technical competency
- Maturity
- Empathy
- Knowledge of pathophysiology of gastrointestinal system
- Physical assessment and screening skills
- Case management skills

RELATED WEBSITES AND PROFESSIONAL ORGANIZATIONS

- American Board of Certification for Gastroenterology Nurses (www.abcgn.org)
- Gastroenterology Nursing (www.gastroenterologynursing.com)
- Society of Gastroenterology Nurses and Associates, Inc. (www.sgna.org)

104 GENERAL PRACTICE NURSE ANESTHETIST

BASIC DESCRIPTION
Nurse anesthetists are responsible for inducing anesthesia, maintaining it at the required levels, and supporting life functions while anesthesia is being administered. Nurse anesthetists administer all types of anesthesia and may perform general, local, and regional anesthesia procedures to pediatric, adult, and geriatric patients, using invasive monitoring techniques when necessary. These nurses practice as part of a highly skilled interdisciplinary team. A variety of practice settings exist including:

- Emergency rooms
- Operating rooms
- Physicians' offices
- Plastic surgery practices
- Dental practices
- Orthopedic practices

EDUCATIONAL REQUIREMENTS
RN preparation with certified registered nurse anesthetist (CRNA) certification is required; a Master of Science in Nursing (MSN) degree is preferred. To enter a nurse anesthetist program, one must possess an active RN license and a baccalaureate degree (may or may not be in nursing). The person must also fulfill certain prerequisites before applying, which vary according to institution. The applicant must also possess a minimum of 1 year of critical care experience as an RN.

CORE COMPETENCIES/SKILLS NEEDED
- Assessment skills and a constant awareness of what is going on at all times
- Skill in history taking and physical assessment
- Patient education skills
- Ability to recognize and take appropriate corrective action (including consulting with anesthesiologist) for abnormal patient responses
- Excellent observation skills
- Ability to provide resuscitative care until the patient has regained control of vital functions
- Skill in administering spinal, epidural, auxiliary, and field blocks

RELATED WEBSITES AND PROFESSIONAL ORGANIZATIONS
- American Association of Nurse Anesthetists (www.aana.com)
- National Board of Recertification for Nurse Anesthetists (www.nbcrna.com)

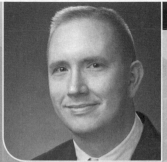

 PROFILE: **CHRISTOPHER REINHART**
Nurse Anesthetist

1. What is your educational background in nursing (and other areas) and what formal credentials do you hold?

I became an RN through a 2-year diploma program. I then earned a Bachelor of Science in Nursing (BSN), MSN with a major in nurse anesthesia, and then a Doctor of Nursing Practice.

I maintain certifications in advanced cardiac life support, pediatric advanced life support, neonatal resuscitation program, basic cardiac life support, and paramedic licensure (EMT-P).

2. How did you first become interested in your current career?

I first became intrigued with nurse anesthesia after meeting a CRNA while I was a nursing student completing my clinical rotations in the operating room. After working in critical care areas for 5 years as an RN, I wanted additional responsibility in a different type of critical care environment. I researched the nurse anesthesia profession, then I interviewed and shadowed several CRNAs before choosing to enter a nurse anesthetist program.

3. What are the most rewarding aspects of your career?

Rewarding aspects of my career include having the ability to calm nervous patients and tend to their needs while they are under anesthesia; being able to relieve a laboring mother's pain through patient education shortly after meeting her, and then administering a spinal or labor epidural; and obtaining respect from my colleagues.

I love doing the job I do, and the results of my work are frequently instantaneous. It is not uncommon to be called to emergency situations anywhere in the hospital to manage an airway or insert a breathing tube to help save a patient's life.

Continued

4. What advice would you give to someone contemplating the same career path in nursing?

If you enjoy working as an RN in the intensive care unit (ICU) or other critical care areas, a career as a CRNA may be for you! The job of a CRNA can be routine at times; however, a patient's condition can deteriorate at a moment's notice requiring critical thinking and rapid interventions from the CRNA.

Admission into CRNA programs is very competitive. Strive to get the highest grade point average possible in your undergraduate preparations. Keep in mind, many hospitals have tuition reimbursement programs for RNs working toward a BSN or MSN. Working in an adult ICU at a larger hospital with high-acuity patients can increase your experience as an RN and improve your chances of getting into a CRNA program. (Some programs accept students from other critical care backgrounds and from small and midsized hospitals as well.) Most CRNA programs currently range from 26 to 30 months of full-time training. The option to train part time does not typically exist. You will have minimal to no time to work as an RN while you are in CRNA training. Therefore, you need to be financially prepared before starting a CRNA program. As CRNA programs continue to transition from the master's degree to the doctorate degree level, training time may be extended.

For additional information, visit the American Association of Nurse Anesthetists website at www.aana.com, and shadow a CRNA.

GENETICS ADVISOR

BASIC DESCRIPTION

A genetics advisor works with patients with, or at risk for, genetic conditions and assists them to promote and maintain wellness. These nurses perform risk assessments and analyze the effect of genetic conditions on health. They provide proper counseling, education, and nursing care to patients affected by genetic diseases. In some cases, they may also be involved in research. Employment opportunities are available in many settings, such as hospitals, schools, business organizations, research centers, and specialty clinics.

EDUCATIONAL REQUIREMENTS

RN preparation with a bachelor's degree in nursing is required. A master's degree in nursing is preferred. Certification is available through the American Nurses Credentialing Center.

CORE COMPETENCIES/SKILLS NEEDED

- Ability to educate patients regarding diagnosis, treatment options, and prognosis
- Sensitivity to patient and family concerns
- Excellent communication and interpersonal skills
- Critical thinking and analytical skills
- Extensive knowledge of genetic conditions

RELATED WEBSITES AND PROFESSIONAL ORGANIZATIONS

- American Board of Genetic Counseling, Inc. (http://www.abgc.net/ABGC/AmericanBoardofGeneticCounselors.asp)
- American Nurses Credentialing Center (www.nursecredentialing.org)
- International Society of Nurses in Genetics (www.isong.org)
- National Society of Genetic Counselors (www.nsgc.org)

106 GENETICS COUNSELOR

BASIC DESCRIPTION

Genetics counselors are nurses or health professionals with specialized graduate degrees and experience in the areas of genetics and counseling. Most enter the field from a variety of disciplines, including biology, genetics, nursing, psychology, public health, and social work. Genetics counselors frequently speak to clients about complex scientific and emotional topics. They work as members of a health care team providing information and support to families who have members with birth defects or genetic disorders and to families who may be at risk for a variety of inherited conditions. Genetics counselors investigate the problem present in the family, interpret information about the disorder, analyze inheritance patterns and risks of recurrence, review available options with the family, serve as patient advocates, and engage in research activities.

EDUCATIONAL REQUIREMENTS

Educational requirements for a genetics counselor would be a master's degree or PhD with advanced education in genetics such as that offered through the National Institutes of Health. The American Board of Genetic Counseling (ABGC) certifies genetic counselors and accredits genetic counseling training programs. Certification in genetic counseling is available through the ABGC. Requirements include documentation of the following: a graduate degree in genetic counseling; clinical experience in an ABGC-approved training site or sites; a log book of 50 supervised cases; and successful completion of both the general and specialty certification examination. Certification for advanced genetics nursing is available through the American Nurses Credentialing Center.

CORE COMPETENCIES/SKILLS NEEDED

- Knowledge of inherited diseases and the ability to counsel parents and families regarding genetic possibilities
- Critical thinking skills
- Collaborative team practice skills
- Deep sensitivity to patient and family concerns
- Listening skills
- Maturity

RELATED WEBSITES AND PROFESSIONAL ORGANIZATIONS

- American Board of Genetic Counseling, Inc. (www.abgc.net/ABGC/AmericanBoardofGeneticCounselors.asp)
- American Nurses Credentialing Center (www.nursecredentialing.org/AdvancedGenetics)
- International Society of Nurses in Genetics (www.isong.org/ISONG_genetic_nurse.php)
- National Society of Genetic Counselors (www.nsgc.org)
- Online Journal of Genetic Counseling (www.nsgc.org/page/journalofgeneticcounseling)

107 GERIATRIC/GERONTOLOGICAL NURSE

BASIC DESCRIPTION

Geriatric or gerontological nurses are RNs who specialize in care of the older adult. Geriatric patients are a unique population with distinctive health considerations because of their advanced age, declining organ functions, and high risk for injury and disease. Geriatric nurses provide nursing care, emotional support to patients and families, and help promote maximum functioning of their patients to enhance quality of life. Job opportunities are found in hospitals, long-term care facilities, home care, skilled nursing facilities, rehabilitation centers, and private practices or clinics. The outlook for positions in gerontology is excellent, as the population of older adults is rapidly increasing.

EDUCATIONAL REQUIREMENTS

RN preparation is required. Basic life support certification is also required. Gerontological nurse certification is encouraged and is available through the American Nurses Credentialing Center.

CORE COMPETENCIES/SKILLS NEEDED

- Ability to provide emotional support
- Thorough knowledge of effects of aging on physiology
- Ability to conduct a complete physical assessment
- Ability to assist patient with activities of daily living
- Ability to collaborate with other members of the health care team
- Compassion and patience

RELATED WEBSITES AND PROFESSIONAL ORGANIZATIONS

- American Nurses Credentialing Center (www.nursecredentialing.org)
- National Gerontological Nursing Association (www.ngna.org)

GERIATRIC NURSE PRACTITIONER

BASIC DESCRIPTION

Geriatric nurse practitioners provide primary and acute care to older persons. They work in hospitals, nursing homes, clinics, home care agencies, senior citizen centers, and in wellness programs in the community.

EDUCATIONAL REQUIREMENTS

RN preparation and a graduate degree from a gerontological nurse practitioner program are required. Certification from the American Nurses Credentialing Center (ANCC) is available. Certification as a gerontology clinical nurse specialist, another advanced nursing practice role, is also available from the ANCC.

CORE COMPETENCIES/SKILLS NEEDED

- Skills in development and implementation of treatment plans for chronic illness
- Ability to provide support, education, and counseling for families
- Understanding of the special needs of the elderly and the process of aging
- Skills in coordination of care

RELATED WEBSITES AND PROFESSIONAL ORGANIZATIONS

- Aging Life Care Association (www.aginglifecare.org)
- American Academy of Nurse Practitioners (www.aanp.org)
- American College of Nurse Practitioners (www.nurse.org/acnp)
- American Nurses Credentialing Center (www.nursecredentialing.org)
- National Gerontological Nursing Association (www.ngna.org)

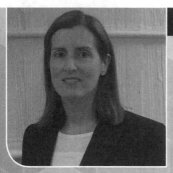

 PROFILE: DONNA E. McCABE

Geriatric Nurse Practitioner, Clinical
Assistant Professor of Nursing

1. What is your educational background in nursing (and other areas) and what formal credentials do you hold?

I have been a nurse for just over 20 years; I am a board-certified geriatric nurse practitioner and have also completed a Doctor of Nursing Practice. In my current full-time role as a clinical assistant professor teaching baccalaureate nursing students, I have the opportunity to share my geriatric nursing expertise. I also have a part-time practice as a geriatric nurse practitioner for a home care agency. I have practiced as a geriatric nurse, nurse leader, and nurse practitioner in hospital, skilled nursing facility, and home care settings. An overarching passion of my career has been an interest in quality and safety as it relates to the health and well-being of older adults.

2. How did you first become interested in your current career?

I am a people person and enjoy being a helping person. I was lucky to be exposed to positive nursing role models in my youth who explained the holistic nature of the profession and the exciting field of geriatric nursing. I became interested in geriatrics early in my career as the population of older adults was growing in the hospital setting. Older adults were in the hospital dealing with the consequences of chronic diseases. My interest in quality and safety was a major factor in leading me along my career path. Nurses were challenged with unique issues of older adults including delirium, falls, and pressure ulcers. I enjoy challenges and wanted to be part of improving systems! I began my education to be a geriatric nurse practitioner 3 years into my career as a nurse and I am currently pursuing a postmaster's degree for a certification as a psychiatric–mental health nurse practitioner to develop my expertise in providing mental health for older adults. I am spurred on by the need to continually improve. Learning never stops!

Continued

PROFILE: DONNA E. McCABE
Continued

3. What are the most rewarding aspects of your career?

The rewarding aspects of my career are many. As a direct care provider, I gain a great deal of satisfaction from helping people live their lives with greater ease. For older adults, particularly those living with chronic disease, specialized appropriate care can add or bring quality to their lives—there is my interest in quality again! As a nurse educator, educating future nurses and health care professionals regarding the special needs of older adults is extremely rewarding. It is a special joy to hear a student or recent graduate nurse tell me that I helped to spark his or her interest in the field.

4. What advice would you give to others contemplating a career such as yours?

I am privileged to often be in a position of giving advice to fledgling nurses. The most sage advice I have to offer is to be a motivated, inquisitive person and do what you love. Students and new nurses sometimes enter school or the profession certain they want to go into a specific specialty. Don't pigeonhole yourself! Explore all the possibilities in nursing; speak with people who work in different areas of the field; and gain experience through volunteering and unconventional avenues.

109   GEROPSYCHIATRIC NURSE

BASIC DESCRIPTION
The geropsychiatric nurse is someone who specializes in caring for older adults with a diagnosis of depression, dementia, and other mental health disorders. These nurses are employed in various health care settings such as home care, ambulatory care settings, and acute care facilities.

EDUCATIONAL REQUIREMENTS
RN preparation and a Bachelor of Science in Nursing are highly preferred. Additional education and training and previous experience in mental health or gerontology are usually required for the position. Basic life support certification is also required.

CORE COMPETENCIES/SKILLS NEEDED
- Knowledge of physiological changes, common pathophysiological disorders, unique needs, psychopharmacology, and behavioral management among older adults
- Excellent communication and assessment skills
- Knowledge of evidence-based information related to the care of older adults who have dementia and other mental health disorders
- Strong analytical and critical thinking skills

RELATED WEBSITES AND PROFESSIONAL ORGANIZATIONS
- American Psychiatric Nurses Association (www.apna.org)
- Hartford Institute for Geriatric Nursing (hartfordign.org/education/geropsych_nursing_comp)

GLOBAL HEALTH NURSE

BASIC DESCRIPTION
Global health nursing is a rapidly growing field that involves international exchange of information regarding nursing practice, health care policies, advancements in education and research, and community outreach in order to improve quality, efficiency, and effectiveness of care across the globe. Nurses play a vital role in the sharing of knowledge to assist other countries in advancing health care delivery to patients. A nurse can be involved in global health nursing in a variety of ways, including being a global nurse consultant, an international nursing educator, a researcher, a philanthropist, founding or leading a global health organization, or volunteering on international medical missions. In many cases, a global nurse will help to advance treatment options and nursing practice in developing countries. A global nurse can create partnerships with nurses in other countries to help improve care delivery globally.

EDUCATIONAL REQUIREMENTS
RN preparation is required. Certificate programs for global health nursing are available and encouraged.

CORE COMPETENCIES/SKILLS NEEDED
- Expert competency in nursing skills and knowledge
- Passion for sharing of information
- Willingness to travel
- Excellent communication and interpersonal skills
- Cultural awareness and sensitivity
- Excellent writing skills
- Ability to work independently and collaborate as a member of a team

RELATED WEBSITES AND PROFESSIONAL ORGANIZATIONS
- Global Nursing Caucus (www.globalnursingcaucus.org)
- International Council of Nurses (www.icn.ch)
- Sigma Theta Tau International (www.nursingsociety.org)
- World Health Organization (www.who.int)

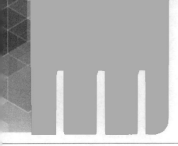

GRANT WRITER

BASIC DESCRIPTION

A grant writer composes applications for funding from private or public sources of support. The monies obtained from a grant are typically given to a business, academic organization, or individual to source a specific project. Development of the grant proposal involves multiple steps: identifying a problem, describing the goals of the project, developing a plan, finding possible funding sources, and writing a proposal. The proposal itself comprises a summary of the problem, a description of the plan, a budgeting plan, and a summary of the qualifications and experience of people who will be involved in the project. There also may be additional attachments, such as letters that support the organization's ability to carry out the project. After the proposal is formatted, edited, and proofed, it is ready for submission.

EDUCATIONAL REQUIREMENTS

A minimum of a bachelor's degree is required, but a master's degree is preferred. Writing experience is required.

CORE COMPETENCIES/SKILLS NEEDED

- Understanding of grantsmanship
- Ability to be highly focused and organized
- Ability to think critically
- Ability to interpret and analyze complex information
- Excellent writing and research skills
- High level of computer literacy
- Knowledge of the research process and potential funding agency requirements
- Ability to work under pressure

RELATED WEBSITE AND PROFESSIONAL ORGANIZATION

- National Institute of Nurse Research; a branch of the U.S. Health and Human Services National Institutes of Health (www.ninr.nih.gov)

HEALTH AND SAFETY MANAGER

BASIC DESCRIPTION

In the role of an administrator, a health and safety manager nurse develops system-wide programs to ensure the delivery of safe and quality care in a health care organization. Using his or her clinical and analytical skills, he or she serves as a consultant and a key management person to administrators in interpreting and analyzing clinical and administrative data.

EDUCATIONAL REQUIREMENTS

RN preparation and master's degree or higher in nursing or a health-related field are required.

CORE COMPETENCIES/SKILLS NEEDED

- At least 5 years of leadership and managerial experience in health care
- Strong communication and interpersonal skills
- Knowledge of risk management and quality improvement principles, The Joint Commission regulations, and safety principles
- Strong skills in data management

RELATED WEBSITE AND PROFESSIONAL ORGANIZATION

- American Organization of Nurse Executives (www.aone.org)

113 HEALTH CARE APPRAISER

BASIC DESCRIPTION
Health care appraisers are professionals who use expertise in health care valuation to serve health care systems and life science organizations. They provide fair market value consultation and analyses for pharmaceuticals and medical equipment for business planning, clinical trials, and data collection. In addition, they can offer support in litigation with valuation analysis as expert witnesses. Clients of a health care appraiser include hospitals, health systems, physicians, outpatient facilities, managed care organizations, nursing homes, pharmaceutical companies, and medical equipment producers.

EDUCATIONAL REQUIREMENTS
A bachelor's degree is required in finance, economics, accounting, or health care. An MBA is preferred. Completion of chartered financial analyst certification, certified valuation analyst credential, certified public accountant certification, and accreditation in business valuation credential are highly recommended. Experience in finance, accounting, health care, or economics work experience is preferred.

CORE COMPETENCIES/SKILLS NEEDED
- Excellent analytical and problem-solving skills
- Ability to understand the details of complex valuation situations
- Knowledge of financial models and financial analysis
- Excellent writing and oral skills
- Excellent computer skills
- Ability to be detail oriented
- Ability to collaborate with multiple disciplines across the executive ladder

RELATED WEBSITE AND PROFESSIONAL ORGANIZATION
- American Society of Appraisers (www.appraisers.org)

HEALTH CARE DISPUTE ANALYST

BASIC DESCRIPTION
Employed in a health care management organization, a health care dispute analyst nurse reviews appeals and billing disputes to ensure that medical claims have been paid correctly. He or she makes recommendations for approval or denial of claims based on assessment and analysis.

EDUCATIONAL REQUIREMENTS
RN preparation is required and a Bachelor of Science in Nursing is highly preferred. Certification in managed care nursing is available from the American Board of Managed Care Nursing.

CORE COMPETENCIES/SKILLS NEEDED
- Understanding of health care payment and reimbursement process
- Knowledge of International Classification of Diseases (ICD-9) codes and experience with Current Procedural Terminology (CPT-4) coding
- Strong computer skills and documentation skills
- Strong organizational skills and ability to work efficiently with multiple documents and data

RELATED WEBSITES AND PROFESSIONAL ORGANIZATIONS
- Aetna Health Organization (www.aetna.com/healthcare-professionals/policies-guidelines/dispute_process.html)
- American Board of Managed Care Nursing (www.abmcn.org)
- Centers for Medicare & Medicaid Services (www.cms.gov/QualityImprovementOrgs/01_Overview.asp)

115 HEALTH CARE MANAGEMENT CONSULTANT

BASIC DESCRIPTION
A health care management consultant can provide many different kinds of services and play a variety of roles. He or she can analyze health care data for businesses, work directly with clients, and consult on information technology projects such as electronic medical record implementation, insurance contract negotiation, clinical improvement plans, and workflow and process design. He or she works as part of an interdisciplinary group to help businesses achieve their health care goals.

EDUCATIONAL REQUIREMENTS
Bachelor's preparation in nursing or in a health care–related field is necessary. A master's degree is preferred. The American Academy of Professional Coders or American Health Information Management Association medical coding certification is also recommended.

CORE COMPETENCIES/SKILLS NEEDED
- Experience in health care and/or project design
- Excellent writing and oral communication skills
- Excellent customer satisfaction skills
- Ability to be highly organized and self-motivated
- Ability to work as part of a team

RELATED WEBSITES AND PROFESSIONAL ORGANIZATIONS
- American Academy of Professional Coders (www.AAPC.com)
- American Health Information Management Association (www.ahima.org)

HEALTH CARE REFORMER

BASIC DESCRIPTION
Health care reform refers to major health policy changes. Nurses can play a big part in health care reform by sharing their expertise and opinions of the health care system and identifying areas that need change or improvement. Opportunities for involvement with health care reform can be obtained by applying for a position within the government; publishing articles or books to share opinions or knowledge; acting as a member, leader, or founder of a committee; or participating in national campaigns to change the health care system.

EDUCATIONAL REQUIREMENTS
There is no educational requirement to be involved in health care reform. To be a well-educated activist for nursing, one should be an RN with a bachelor's degree in nursing.

CORE COMPETENCIES/SKILLS NEEDED
- Excellent communication skills
- Leadership skills
- Dedication and passion for the cause
- Ability to professionally voice an opinion
- Persistence, courage, and patience
- Creativity and ability to think critically
- Knowledge of state and federal laws that affect health care and political and legislative procedures
- Knowledge of the health system

RELATED WEBSITES AND PROFESSIONAL ORGANIZATIONS
- Institute for Healthcare Improvement (www.ihi.org)
- www.HealthCare.gov (federal government website managed by the Centers for Medicare & Medicaid Services)

117 HEALTH CARE REPORTER/JOURNALIST

BASIC DESCRIPTION
Nurses who have an interest in publishing or writing can become reporters or journalists. Their role is to increase the public's awareness of health care news and issues through the written and spoken word. There are a variety of career paths in health care journalism, such as working as a news reporter/broadcast journalist, journal editor, health care policy analyst, or a writer. Employment can be found within a health care journal, newspaper, news station, nonprofit organization, or websites.

EDUCATIONAL REQUIREMENTS
Bachelor's degree in journalism, English, or a health care–related field is required.

CORE COMPETENCIES/SKILLS NEEDED
- Awareness of health care news and issues
- Experience with computers and digital media
- Expert level writing skills
- Excellent communication skills
- Fast learner and ability to meet tight deadlines
- Advanced problem-solving and critical thinking skills
- Ability to work well under pressure
- Ability to be organized and detail oriented
- Outgoing personality with excellent people skills

RELATED WEBSITE AND PROFESSIONAL ORGANIZATION
- Association of Health Care Journalists (www.healthjournalism.org)

HEALTH CARE RISK MANAGER

BASIC DESCRIPTION

Health care risk managers are responsible for managing actual and potential risk in a health care organization to ensure quality patient care. They work closely with hospital administrators to manage liability by developing and implementing policies and protocols that improve patient safety. They may also work with the legal department to address medical malpractice or worker's compensation cases. Education and training of staff members and addressing patient complaints may also be included in job responsibilities. Employment can be found in hospitals, health systems, rehabilitation centers, and clinics.

EDUCATIONAL REQUIREMENTS

A bachelor's degree in a health care–related field is required. In some cases, a master's degree in a health care–related field is required. RN preparation is not required, but is an excellent educational background for risk management.

CORE COMPETENCIES/SKILLS NEEDED
- Knowledge of government regulations
- Thorough understanding of organization's policies and procedures
- Strong writing skills
- Excellent verbal and written communication skills
- Strong assessment skills
- Strong leadership and management skills
- Ability to be organized and attentive to detail
- Ability to analyze complex situations
- Ability to handle stress and difficult decisions

RELATED WEBSITES AND PROFESSIONAL ORGANIZATIONS
- Agency for Healthcare Research and Quality (www.ahrq.gov)
- American Society for Healthcare Risk Management (www.ashrm.org)
- Risk Management Society (www.rims.org)
- The Joint Commission (www.jointcommission.org)

119 HEALTH CARE SURVEYOR

BASIC DESCRIPTION
A health care surveyor nurse is responsible for ensuring that health care providers and health care agencies meet state and federal statutes and regulations. Responsibilities may include surveying health care agencies, investigating complaints against health care professionals and health care agencies, auditing Medicaid claims, and participating in disaster or health care emergencies.

EDUCATIONAL REQUIREMENTS
A Bachelor of Science in Nursing degree is required; a master's degree is preferred. Current RN license and successful completion of prerequisite training course within the first year of employment are required.

CORE COMPETENCIES/SKILLS NEEDED
- Willingness to travel, and flexibility with time
- Extensive knowledge of state and federal health care standards and regulations
- Basic computer skills
- Excellent writing and interpersonal communication skills
- Ability to work with members of the health care team

RELATED WEBSITE AND PROFESSIONAL ORGANIZATION
- State Department of Health

HEALTH CENTER NURSE

BASIC DESCRIPTION
The health center nurse provides a comprehensive range of services to individuals and families ranging from conducting a health history and health screening; assisting physicians and other health care providers with procedures; administering treatments, immunizations, and medications per physician's orders; and maintaining charts and ensuring proper documentation. The health center nurse may also be required to take an active role in cases of public health emergency. These nurses works in ambulatory centers, home care agencies, or public health organizations.

EDUCATIONAL REQUIREMENTS
RN preparation is required; basic life support certification is required.

CORE COMPETENCIES/SKILLS NEEDED
- Strong assessment and analytical skills
- Strong computer and documentation skills
- Flexibility, assertiveness, and creativity
- Excellent interpersonal and communication skills
- Knowledge of public health laws
- Ability to work with other members of the health care team
- Ability to assume managerial responsibilities if working in ambulatory centers

RELATED WEBSITE AND PROFESSIONAL ORGANIZATION
- National Association of Community Health Centers (www.nachc.org)

121 HEALTH COACH

BASIC DESCRIPTION
Health coaches are primarily RNs, but also respiratory therapists and dieticians, who work with patients around the clock offering services completely by telephone. They provide state-of-the-art health information and a calming voice when a patient is having a crisis or is in pain or indecision, and provide tips on self-care. Health coaches stay in contact with their patients and provide information and support until patients begin to feel better and gain confidence. Coaches have more time with patients to provide them with new tools and more support, thereby helping them understand their conditions better and navigate their way through the health care system. Patients will sometimes reveal things over the phone that they would not say in person, fostering deep interactions with their health coach. A large part of health coaching is encouraging patients to become actively involved in their own health and to work with their health care providers in making critical health decisions. Patients are also encouraged to manage their health conditions in ways that reflect the patients' personal values and preferences. Health coaches generally work for independent companies; they also may be independent consultants.

EDUCATIONAL REQUIREMENTS
RN preparation is required.

CORE COMPETENCIES/SKILLS NEEDED
- Excellent listening and interpersonal skills based on the fact that all services are telephone based
- Extensive clinical knowledge
- Knowledge of health promotion, illness prevention, and treatment
- Counseling skills

RELATED WEBSITES AND PROFESSIONAL ORGANIZATIONS
- Georgetown University Certificate in Health Coaching (http://scs.georgetown.edu/programs/385/health-coaching)
- National Society of Health Coaches (www.nshcoa.com)

HEALTH POLICY ANALYST

BASIC DESCRIPTION

A health policy analyst collects data and conducts background research, synthesizes research findings, and reports this information in verbal or written formats, usually on a particular project that serves the client's needs. Because of the analyst's knowledge of health and health care, the data and background documents are framed to convey information about the broad determinants of health and the impact of the data on policy change. Health policy analysts may be independent consultants or may be employed by professional organizations. Health policy analysts may be employed by government agencies (e.g., state or city health departments).

EDUCATIONAL REQUIREMENTS

RN preparation is required; a Master of Science in Nursing and Master of Public Health or equivalent are desired.

CORE COMPETENCIES/SKILLS NEEDED

- Legislative background
- Analytical skills in public health and health care issues
- Knowledge of political and legislative processes
- Appropriate research skills to seek a variety of data sources, and to prioritize among the data sources for accuracy and bias
- Excellent and accurate attention to detail in all written and verbal communication
- Ability to effectively prioritize project tasks and schedules
- Broad knowledge of key processes related to legislation, regulation, and politics on the local, state, and legislative levels
- Ability to extract and summarize large amounts of data and evidence to support health policies

RELATED WEBSITE AND PROFESSIONAL ORGANIZATION

- American Association of Colleges of Nursing (www.aacn.nche.edu/government-affairs/AACNPolicyHandbook_2010.pdf)

123 HERBALIST

BASIC DESCRIPTION
The herbalist nurse assists patients in the proper and safe use of herbal medicine in the patient medical care regimen especially when used with pharmaceutical agents. Herbalist RNs combine their knowledge of nursing and herbal medicine to design individualized treatment plans.

EDUCATIONAL REQUIREMENTS
RN preparation and advanced education on herbal medicine are required.

CORE COMPETENCIES/SKILLS NEEDED
- Advanced knowledge of herbal medicine
- Strong knowledge of pharmacokinetics and pharmacodynamics
- Excellent interpersonal communication skills

RELATED WEBSITES AND PROFESSIONAL ORGANIZATIONS
- American Botanical Council (abc.herbalgram.org/site/PageServer?pagename=Homepage)
- American Herbal Products Association (www.ahpa.org)

HISTORIAN

BASIC DESCRIPTION
The nurse historian documents and identifies the dilemmas with which nursing has struggled through time. History provides current nurses with the same intellectual and political tools that determined nursing pioneers applied to shape nursing values and beliefs to the social context of their times. Nursing history includes the study of labor history, gender studies, oral and social history, anthropology, and the social sciences. Such study exposes nursing students, practitioners, faculty, and administrators to the helpfulness of using history to understand the evolution of the profession. It provides a historical perspective to debates on health policy, encourages reflective practice among nursing professionals, and provides the historical legacy of the profession. Nurse historians are most often employed by academic institutions and the historical research is completed as part of their scholarship.

EDUCATIONAL REQUIREMENTS
A PhD is required to do the historical research and to hold a university faculty position as a nurse historian.

CORE COMPETENCIES/SKILLS NEEDED
- Interest in doing historical research and teaching
- Ability to attend to details
- Skills in historical research methods

RELATED WEBSITES AND PROFESSIONAL ORGANIZATIONS
- American Association for the History of Nursing (www.aahn.org)
- Barbara Bates Center for the Study of the History of Nursing (www.nursing .upenn.edu/history)

125 HIV/AIDS SPECIALIST

BASIC DESCRIPTION
An HIV/AIDS specialist is a nurse who works primarily with patients inflicted with HIV/AIDS. HIV/AIDS specialists may work in acute care facilities, long-term care facilities, home care, and hospice.

EDUCATIONAL REQUIREMENTS
RN preparation is required. Palliative care certification is available, but not always required for job placement; certification by the Association of Nurses in AIDS Care or HIV/AIDS Nursing Certification Board is available as an AIDS certified RN or advanced AIDS certified RN.

CORE COMPETENCIES/SKILLS NEEDED
- Expertise in caring for those who have HIV/AIDS
- Extensive knowledge of HIV/AIDS disease process
- Knowledge of death, dying, and grieving process
- Skills to provide counseling to families of those inflicted with HIV/AIDS
- Ability to care, manage, and teach those inflicted
- Assessment skills for pain and pain management techniques
- Knowledge and understanding of the ethical issues that arise at the end of life

RELATED WEBSITES AND PROFESSIONAL ORGANIZATIONS
- Association of Nurses in AIDS Care (www.anacnet.org)
- HIV/AIDS Nursing Certification Board (www.hancb.org/Index/index.php)
- World Homecare and Hospice Organization (www.whho.org)

HOLISTIC HEALTH NURSE

BASIC DESCRIPTION
Holistic nursing involves all aspects of wellness and healing of a holistic nature, with holism defined as the mind–body–spirit connection. Holistic nurses treat the whole person, not just a disease or symptom. Working as a holistic nurse is a chance to be a part of a growing specialty, but because the field is new, some skepticism still exists. Opportunities for employment exist in health care facilities, holistic health and wellness centers, spas and health clubs, private practices, and pain management centers.

EDUCATIONAL REQUIREMENTS
RN preparation is required. Certification in holistic nursing is available from the American Holistic Nurses Credentialing Corporation.

CORE COMPETENCIES/SKILLS NEEDED
- Interest in—and commitment to focus on—wellness, healing, and illness prevention from a more spiritual and natural perspective
- Commitment to a holistic philosophy
- Knowledge of complementary and alternative therapies
- Openness to go beyond the conventions of traditional medicine and health care

RELATED WEBSITES AND PROFESSIONAL ORGANIZATIONS
- American Holistic Nurses Association (www.ahna.org)
- American Holistic Nurses Credentialing Corporation (www.ahncc.org)

127

HOME HEALTH CARE NURSE PRACTITIONER

BASIC DESCRIPTION

Home health care nurse practitioners provide home-based care to chronically ill patients across age groups. They conduct assessment, diagnose disease conditions, order and provide treatment, and evaluate patient care. They also provide referral services if necessary. They work with members of the health care team and maintain close communication with patients and caregivers.

EDUCATIONAL REQUIREMENTS

RN preparation, a master's degree, and nurse practitioner certification are required.

CORE COMPETENCIES/SKILLS NEEDED

- Excellent assessment and analytical skills
- Ability to work independently
- Knowledge of home health care regulations and reimbursement
- Excellent organizational, leadership, and communication skills
- Knowledge of regulations on advance directives and end-of-life care

RELATED WEBSITES AND PROFESSIONAL ORGANIZATIONS

- American College of Nurse Practitioners (www.acnpweb.org/i4a/pages/index.cfm?pageid=1)
- National Association for Home Care & Hospice (www.nahc.org)
- Visiting Nurse Service of New York (www.vnsny.org)

HOME HEALTH NURSE

128

BASIC DESCRIPTION

A home health nurse provides nursing care and support to individuals and families in their own homes, assisted living facilities, or nursing homes. This care may be provided before or after acute and long-term illness. Home health nurses may be prepared as generalists for care of all patients or may be specialists (e.g., oncology or geriatric nurses). Home health nurses provide direct patient care in contrast to public or community health nurses whose focus is population based.

EDUCATIONAL REQUIREMENTS

RN preparation is required.

CORE COMPETENCIES/SKILLS NEEDED

- Ability to function independently at an optimal level
- Excellent communication and bedside manner with patients and their families
- Ability to perceive the patient's needs in relation to the home environment
- Ability to conform and adapt traditional nursing care to the home environment
- Knowledge of many cultures and openness to work with people from a wide variety of cultures
- Excellent assessment skills
- Autonomy and flexibility

RELATED WEBSITES AND PROFESSIONAL ORGANIZATIONS

- Home Healthcare Nurses Association (hhna.org)
- National Association for Home Care & Hospice (www.nahc.org)
- Visiting Nurse Associations of America (www.vnaa.org)

129 HOSPICE AND PALLIATIVE CARE NURSE

BASIC DESCRIPTION

Hospice and palliative care nurses work with people who have terminal illnesses and are predicted to die within 6 months. Hospice or palliative care can take place in a hospice facility, but approximately 90% of patients receive care at home or in other residential care institutions. Nurses who work with dying patients and their loved ones must be able to manage dealing with death on a daily basis; the stress of the work requires maturity.

EDUCATIONAL REQUIREMENTS

RN preparation is required. Usually 1 to 2 years of experience in home care and oncology is recommended before entering this specialty. Certification in various roles is available in this specialty—as a Certified Hospice and Palliative Care Nurse (CHPN)—through the National Board for Certification of Hospice and Palliative Nurses.

CORE COMPETENCIES/SKILLS NEEDED

- Attention to the psychological, spiritual, physical, and social aspects of care as related to the patient's quality of life
- Skill in using resources found within the home or other residential site to provide end-of-life nursing care
- Ability to provide stress relief for dying patients and their families
- Skill in relieving multiple physical symptoms such as pain, dyspnea, fatigue, anorexia, and delirium
- Skill in helping patients deal with emotional symptoms such as depression, anxiety, and fear associated with facing impending death
- Collaboration with other members of the interdisciplinary team to help relieve patient suffering

RELATED WEBSITES AND PROFESSIONAL ORGANIZATIONS

- Center to Advance Palliative Care (www.capc.org/providers/palliative-care-resources/palliative-care-resources-certification-licensing)
- End-of-Life Nursing Education Consortium (www.aacn.nche.edu/elnec)
- Hospice and Palliative Nurses Association (www.hpna.org)
- Hospice Foundation of America (hospicefoundation.org)
- World Homecare and Hospice Organization (www.whho.org)

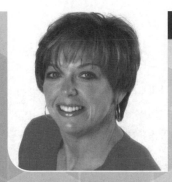

 PROFILE: MALENE DAVIS
Hospice Nurse

1. What is your educational background in nursing (and other areas) and what formal credentials do you hold?

I am an RN and hold a Bachelor of Science in Nursing, a Master of Science in Nursing, and an MBA. I am also a CHPN.

2. How did you first become interested in your current career?

I began as a nurse in oncology and was initially very interested in the science behind treating cancer and serious diseases. Over time, as I watched patients experience the pain and difficult symptoms associated with a lot of advanced medical treatments, I found that it was critical to provide holistic care, not only by offering compassion, but also by offering pain relief and symptom management.

This experience coupled with my personal encounter with hospice—when my ill grandmother just wanted to "go home"—compelled me to found the nonprofit Hospice Care Corporation in Arthurdale, West Virginia, in 1988, which has become the largest hospice program in the state. I started it from the ground up! My next personal encounter was in 1998, when my beloved father was dying.

3. What are the most rewarding aspects of your career?

I have been actively promoting palliative and hospice care for most of my career. The most rewarding aspect of this has been leading a movement that, over time, will enhance the lives of thousands of patients and families who are coping with advanced illnesses. As our nation's aging population surges, the need for coordinated, holistic care will become that much more relevant. I can't think of a better job to have than to promote this type of care so that Americans from coast to coast have dignity and comfort in the face of serious illness.

Continued

PROFILE: MALENE DAVIS
Continued

4. What advice would you give to someone contemplating the same career path in nursing?

Nursing is, first and foremost, about providing excellent clinical care and compassion to people who are sick. If you have a desire to do that and to do more than that, as I have done, opportunities abound. This is particularly true as our country reexamines the current health care system and looks for better ways to improve medical care. The simple truth is we need good nurses. They are the backbone of our health system. If you feel this is your calling, I encourage you to pursue nursing with verve and vigor. Your efforts will pay off!

HOSPITAL BED MANAGEMENT DIRECTOR

BASIC DESCRIPTION

A hospital bed management director is responsible for overseeing appropriate bed assignment to inpatients. He or she works very closely with hospital leadership from nursing, environmental services, transport services, and case management to coordinate timely throughput of patients. He or she works to create and implement policies and protocols to promote proactive discharges, plans for hospital overcrowding, and anticipates hospital admissions and transfers to ensure effective patient flow. He or she must closely monitor hospital capacity and strategize solutions to throughput issues.

EDUCATIONAL REQUIREMENTS

A bachelor's degree in nursing, business, or a health care–related field is required. A master's degree in business or health care is preferred. Relevant clinical experience is desirable.

CORE COMPETENCIES/SKILLS NEEDED

- High organization skills
- Excellent leadership and managerial skills
- Ability to give direction and delegate
- An eye for detail
- Excellent oral and written communication
- Ability to collaborate
- Understanding of necessary bed attributes for patient needs
- Knowledge of organizational bed allotment for levels of care

RELATED WEBSITES AND PROFESSIONAL ORGANIZATIONS

There are no related websites or organizations.

131 HOSPITAL/HEALTH SYSTEM CHIEF EXECUTIVE OFFICER

BASIC DESCRIPTION
A health system chief executive officer (CEO) is the highest-ranking executive officer in an institution that delivers health care. The CEO is responsible for making administrative and organizational decisions to ultimately ensure that the needs of the company, employees, and clients are met in an efficient, financially sound, and effective manner. Other duties include setting and maintaining the company's mission, vision, and culture; building and managing the senior leadership team; evaluating and analyzing company performance; and strategizing financial decisions.

EDUCATIONAL REQUIREMENTS
A bachelor's degree in nursing or another health care–related field is necessary. A master's degree in nursing, business administration, or health care administration is also required. A doctoral prepared candidate is highly desirable. Certification as a nurse executive is available through American Nurses Credentialing Center.

CORE COMPETENCIES/SKILLS NEEDED
- Excellent leadership and management skills
- Assertiveness, resilience, and decisiveness
- Ability to work independently or collaboratively and delegate tasks as needed
- Skill in using technology
- Strong clinical knowledge and skills
- Ability to analyze, interpret, and utilize data in decision making
- Excellent leadership and management skills
- Assertiveness, objectivity, and ability to make important decisions under pressure
- Strong communication and interpersonal skills
- Willingness to take risks
- Knowledge of business and financial skills

RELATED WEBSITES AND PROFESSIONAL ORGANIZATIONS
- American College of Healthcare Executives (www.ache.org)
- American Hospital Association (www.aha.org)
- American Nurses Credentialing Center (www.nursecredentialing.org)
- American Organization of Nurse Executives (www.aone.org)
- Institute for Healthcare Improvement (www.ihi.org)

HOSPITAL/HEALTH SYSTEM CHIEF OPERATING OFFICER

132

BASIC DESCRIPTION

A hospital or health system chief operating officer (COO) is the executive leader who is responsible for managing and directing all business operations. This individual reports to the chief executive officer. The COO ensures smooth operations through direction, evaluation, and coordination among several departments within the hospital or health system, including process improvement initiatives, clinical outcomes, standardization of operations, patient satisfaction, and resource utilization. He or she must ensure that the mission and vision of an organization are met through task execution.

EDUCATIONAL REQUIREMENTS

A minimum of a master's degree in a health care or health care administration field is required. A doctorate level degree is highly desirable. Certification is available through American College of Healthcare Executives or American Organization of Nurse Executives.

CORE COMPETENCIES/SKILLS NEEDED

- Excellent leadership and communication skills
- Assertiveness, resilience, and decisiveness
- Strong interpersonal skills
- Willingness to take risks
- Knowledge of business and financial skills
- Ability to work independently or collaboratively and delegate tasks as needed
- Skill in using technology
- Strong clinical skills and knowledge
- Ability to multitask
- Ability to analyze, interpret, and utilize data in decision making
- Current knowledge of regulatory standards
- Ability to be organized and detail oriented
- Ability to identify needs for change and develop process improvements to achieve positive change
- Ability to build strong relationships within and outside of the organization

RELATED WEBSITES AND PROFESSIONAL ORGANIZATIONS

- American College of Healthcare Executives (www.ache.org)
- American Hospital Association (www.aha.org)
- American Nurses Credentialing Center (www.nursecredentialing.org)
- American Organization of Nurse Executives (www.aone.org)
- Institute for Healthcare Improvement (www.ihi.org)

HOSPITAL ORIENTATION EDUCATOR

BASIC DESCRIPTION
Hospital orientation educators specialize in preparing newly hired employees at a health care organization for their new jobs. They educate the new employees on institutional policies and protocols, familiarize them with the mission and vision of the organization, teach skills for hospital-specific equipment or technologies, and provide them with the necessary general information to function in their positions.

EDUCATIONAL REQUIREMENTS
RN preparation is required. A master's degree in nursing or education is usually required. Certification as a nurse educator is available through the National League for Nursing.

CORE COMPETENCIES/SKILLS NEEDED
- Knowledge of teaching/learning and/or management principles and practices
- Time management skills
- Ability to work independently or as part of a team
- Research and/or publication skills
- Motivational and mentoring skills
- Well versed in the organization's policies, procedures, mission, and values
- Excellent verbal communication skills
- Innovativeness and high energy
- Strong interpersonal skills

RELATED WEBSITE AND PROFESSIONAL ORGANIZATION
- National League for Nursing (www.nln.org)

134 HYPERBARIC NURSE

BASIC DESCRIPTION
A hyperbaric nurse is a highly specialized nurse who cares for patients in hyperbaric or decompression chambers. These chambers are used to care for a specific population of patients who require certain atmospheric pressures for effective therapy. A hyperbaric nurse is responsible for delivery of safe, quality care while functioning as a clinician, educator, researcher, and/or manager.

EDUCATIONAL REQUIREMENTS
RN preparation is required. Certification is available through the National Board of Diving & Hyperbaric Medical Technology.

CORE COMPETENCIES/SKILLS NEEDED
- Knowledge of diseases that require treatment through hyperbaric chambers and the altered environment of care in a hyperbaric treatment
- Knowledge of risks involved in hyperbaric chambers

RELATED WEBSITES AND ORGANIZATIONS
- Baromedical Nurses Association (www.hyperbaricnurses.org)
- National Board of Diving & Hyperbaric Medical Technology (www.nbdhmt.org)

BASIC DESCRIPTION

An industrial nurse is a registered nurse who oversees safety and medical needs of workers in an industrial setting. Job responsibilities may include intervening during work-related illness or injury, making referrals to a higher level of care as needed, managing employee health status information, managing workers' compensation cases, and facilitating workplace safety.

EDUCATIONAL REQUIREMENTS

RN preparation is required. Basic life support certification is also required. Certification through the American Board for Occupational Health Nurses is encouraged.

CORE COMPETENCIES/SKILLS NEEDED

- Management and communication skills
- Basic computer skills
- Crisis intervention and ability to treat work-related injuries
- Ability to create and maintain a safe work environment

RELATED WEBSITES AND PROFESSIONAL ORGANIZATIONS

- American Board for Occupational Health Nurses, Inc. (www.abohn.org)
- Occupational Safety and Health Administration (www.osha.gov)

136 INFECTION CONTROL NURSE

BASIC DESCRIPTION
An infection control nurse is one who specializes in identifying, controlling, and preventing outbreaks of infection in health care settings and the community. These nurses establish and implement guidelines directed toward the prevention, detection, and control of infectious processes. Activities include collection and analysis of infection control data; planning, implementation, and evaluation of infection prevention and control measures; education of individuals about infection risk, prevention, and control; development and revision of infection control policies and procedures; investigation of suspected outbreaks of infection; and provision of consultation on infection risk assessment, prevention, and control strategies. Practice areas include long-term care facilities, community or regional hospitals, nonacute inpatient institutions, industry, private and public settings, nursing homes, and mental health facilities.

EDUCATIONAL REQUIREMENTS
RN preparation and a Bachelor of Science in Nursing are required. Documented educational programs related to epidemiology, sterilization, sanitation, disinfection, patient care practice, and adult education principles are a requirement. Certification as an infection control practitioner is preferred and is available from the Certification Board of Infection Control and Epidemiology, Inc.; a Master of Science in Nursing or Master of Public Health may be required.

CORE COMPETENCIES/SKILLS NEEDED
- Ability to diagnose HIV/AIDS, tuberculosis, scabies, nosocomial infections, and other infectious diseases
- Knowledge of prevention of infectious diseases
- Knowledge and expertise in microbiology, epidemiology, statistics, sterilization and disinfection, infectious diseases, and antibiotic usage
- Consultative and teaching skills
- Knowledge of the multitude of federal and organizational mandates

RELATED WEBSITES AND PROFESSIONAL ORGANIZATIONS
- Association for Professionals in Infection Control and Epidemiology, Inc. (www.apic.org)
- Centers for Disease Control and Prevention (www.cdc.gov)
- Certification Board of Infection Control and Epidemiology, Inc. (www.cbic.org)

INFECTION CONTROL OFFICER

137

BASIC DESCRIPTION

An infection control officer is a health care professional assigned to a department or division to ensure that proper infection control procedures and practices are being carried out per institutional policy. Infection control officers are responsible for environmental appropriateness, communication with safety officers, and response to infectious exposures within the organization. They must also respond to infectious breakouts or exposure incidents that occur to ensure that appropriate documentation and treatment are completed. They can also act as resources and educators for staff.

EDUCATIONAL REQUIREMENTS

RN preparation is required. A bachelor's degree in nursing is required with relevant clinical experience. Certification is available.

CORE COMPETENCIES/SKILLS NEEDED

- Knowledge of communicable diseases and evidence-based infectious control practices
- Excellent communication and leadership skills
- Attention to detail
- Ability to interpret and report data
- Ability to work independently or as part of a team
- Knowledge of emergency management
- Ability to advocate for patients and staff

RELATED WEBSITES AND PROFESSIONAL ORGANIZATIONS

- Centers for Disease Control and Prevention (www.cdc.gov)
- Certification Board of Infection Control and Epidemiology, Inc. (www.cbic.org)

138 INFECTIOUS DISEASE NURSE PRACTITIONER

BASIC DESCRIPTION
Infectious disease nurse practitioners work across all health care settings to prevent, manage, and treat infectious diseases. They can serve as educators, health policy makers and advocates, direct care providers, or researchers.

EDUCATIONAL REQUIREMENTS
RN preparation, master's degree, and certification in infection control are required.

CORE COMPETENCIES/SKILLS NEEDED
- Knowledge of epidemiology and statistics
- Knowledge of health policy impacting infection control and risk assessment
- Excellent verbal and written communication skills
- Strong computer and interpersonal skills
- Ability to work in a team

RELATED WEBSITES AND PROFESSIONAL ORGANIZATIONS
- Association of Professionals in Infection Control and Epidemiology (www.apic.org)
- Centers for Disease Control and Prevention (www.cdc.gov)
- Certification Board of Infection Control and Epidemiology, Inc. (www.cbic.org)

INFORMATICIST

BASIC DESCRIPTION
A nurse informaticist is an RN who works to integrate information technology with nursing practice. Nurse informaticists utilize health information technologies to improve communication, advance patient care, support health care professionals, and manage information. They work to develop, implement, improve, or educate providers regarding technological applications in health care. In addition, they collect data and conduct research to improve processes.

EDUCATIONAL REQUIREMENTS
RN preparation with a minimum of a bachelor's degree is needed to be a nurse informaticist; however, a master's degree in nursing informatics is preferred. Experience working with health information technology is essential. Informatics nursing certification is available through the American Nurses Credentialing Center.

CORE COMPETENCIES/SKILLS NEEDED
- Experience working with and extensive knowledge of electronic medical records and applications of health information technology
- Ability to take initiative and work independently
- Ability to conduct major analyses of information
- Skills in developing data analyses systems and methodologies
- Good communication and analytical skills
- Experience in patient care
- Marketing skills
- Ability to work efficiently and individually or as part of a team

RELATED WEBSITES AND PROFESSIONAL ORGANIZATIONS
- American Medical Informatics Association: Nursing Informatics Working Group (www.amia.org/programs/working-groups/nursing-informatics)
- American Nursing Credentialing Center (www.nursecredentialing.org)
- American Nursing Informatics Association (www.ania.org)

140 INFORMATICS SPECIALIST

BASIC DESCRIPTION
Informatics nursing is the integration of nursing and its information management with information processing and communication technology to support the health of people worldwide. Nursing informatics is the specialty that integrates science, computer science, and information science in identifying, collecting, processing, and managing data and information to support nursing practice, administration, research, and the expansion of nursing knowledge. Nursing informatics is considered by many executives as a way to improve quality of care and reduce excess expenditures. Informatics nurses work in a variety of settings such as hospitals, clinics, educational settings, and private consulting firms.

EDUCATIONAL REQUIREMENTS
A Bachelor of Science in Nursing (BSN) degree is required; a master's degree in nursing informatics is preferred. Credentialing is available through the American Nurses Credentialing Center.

CORE COMPETENCIES/SKILLS NEEDED
- Ability to conduct major analyses of information
- Skill in developing data analysis systems and methodologies
- Consultation skills regarding the use of technology
- Marketing skills
- Skill in developing and disseminating reports to staff about cost and other trends in health care
- Ability to use various resources to analyze and interpret variances and make comparisons with national and regional benchmarks
- Ability to manage multiple priorities
- Ability to work independently

RELATED WEBSITES AND PROFESSIONAL ORGANIZATIONS
- American Nurses Credentialing Center (www.nursingworld.org)
- American Nursing Informatics Association (www.ania.org)

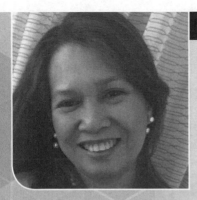

 PROFILE: **MARY JOY GARCIA-DIA**
Informatics Specialist

1. What is your educational background in nursing (and other areas) and what formal credentials do you hold?

I received a BSN, a master's degree in nursing informatics, and completed my doctoral program (DNP), with a leadership track. I have more than 14 years of clinical nursing experience, as well as 12 years of health care informatics experience, which includes teaching and information technology (IT) work. As part of my work experience, I was trained and certified in systems configuration of various clinical systems and the electronic medical record.

2. How did you first become interested in your current career?

As a critical care nurse working in an intensive care unit in 1990, I was fascinated by how data was captured from the monitors and ventilators and fed into the electronic record. All nursing documentation was entered electronically, from admission assessment to vital signs, intake and output flowsheet, medication administration records, fall and neurological assessments, and daily nursing notes. The critical care system allowed nurses to calculate drips, and we could map the vital signs and correlate how well the patient was responding to the IV medications to maintain and monitor hemodynamic status as it related to laboratory results. The seamless integration led me to inquire how this data transfer was programmed. A new field, called "informatics" by *U.S. News & World Report*, was being described that would change health care delivery through automation. A great opportunity presented itself while I was researching this field—New York University offered a new master's program in nursing informatics. I switched my course from Master of Public Heath to Informatics. That was the best professional and academic decision that I made for my career.

Continued

3. What are the most rewarding aspects of your career?

Being on the cusp of changes in technology and the health care industry as an informatics specialist is an exciting and mind-expanding experience. I am exposed to technology solutions (wireless, biosensors, data exchange and integration, simulations, and augmented reality) that can transform the clinician's workflow, and improve business processes and patient quality outcomes. This is the opportunity that excites me the most, which leads to the innovative and critical aspects of my work: blending and integrating these technologies to match how we provide care to our patients while staying close to the overarching goal of meeting both clinical and operational needs of our clinicians. When clinicians are able to have the decision support needed to provide safe, quality care and engage with our patients to understand and take control of their own health data, then I know that I am making a difference in improving health, eliminating medical errors, and reducing costs. Through working with various IT teams, we empower providers and patients to trust the accuracy of health data and information so both can work positively in understanding the disease process, looking into treatment options, and correlating that data in predicting the best outcomes based on the individual patient's plan of care. The meaningful use of data in both clinical and research settings is the ultimate benefit and value that we as informatics specialists provide. But we have a bigger role to play in today's innovative health care industry. It is this direction that I think will have a huge impact and greater reward as we continue to expand the role of clinical informatics toward predictive modeling, population health, and health information exchange.

4. What advice would you give to someone contemplating the same career path in nursing?

My advice to people who are interested in the field of informatics is to follow their passion. The work that comes with being an informatics specialist is not for the faint of heart. As in any specialized field, one has to stay resilient to overcome the barriers that come with being a minority among coworkers in a highly technical work environment. It is important to remember that clinical skills and nursing experience are not easily learned or acquired by a technical person. Be proud of who you are as a registered nurse because regardless of where you work—for a health care organization, as a consultant, or with a vendor—you are the link and advocate in ensuring that safe, quality processes are in place for patients and clinicians before these systems and networks are implemented and used within the environment of care.

INFUSION THERAPY NURSE

BASIC DESCRIPTION

An infusion nurse has expertise in the field of infusion therapy. The infusion nurse's role is to perform intravenous therapy, as well as patient education regarding the task being performed. There are opportunities for infusion therapy nurses to work in hospitals, home care, and various alternative settings, such as hospice or long-term care facilities.

EDUCATIONAL REQUIREMENTS

RN preparation is required. Certification is available from the Infusion Nurses Certification Corporation.

CORE COMPETENCIES/SKILLS NEEDED

- Skill in venipuncture
- Knowledge of ways to ensure quality care to patients
- Knowledge of nosocomial infection rates and prevention
- Good interpersonal skills

RELATED WEBSITE AND PROFESSIONAL ORGANIZATION

- Infusion Nurses Society (www.ins1.org)

142 INTAKE NURSE

BASIC DESCRIPTION
Intake registered nurses are sometimes the first health care professionals whom patients meet in the acute care setting. Their responsibilities may include conducting an initial assessment and obtaining nursing history for newly admitted patients. Aside from providing patients with an overview of the unit, they may also determine the types and intensity of services that patients will receive in a particular unit.

EDUCATIONAL REQUIREMENTS
In hospitals that have a specific job description for this role, a Bachelor of Science in Nursing is highly preferred and several years of acute care experience is a requirement.

CORE COMPETENCIES/SKILLS NEEDED
- Good assessment, triage, and interview skills
- Excellent communication skills and knowledge of specific services in the hospital
- Excellent organization skills and basic computer skills
- Ability to work in a fast-paced environment

RELATED WEBSITES AND PROFESSIONAL ORGANIZATIONS
There are no related websites or organizations.

INTERNATIONAL HEALTH NURSE

BASIC DESCRIPTION

International health nurses may work on a wide range of global health issues in a number of settings. They may be employed by governmental agencies (e.g., the United Nations, the World Health Organization, or nongovernmental organizations). They also could be independent consultants. The topics of importance to global nursing include the increasing disparity in access to health care; the growing population of the poor (more than 1 billion people do not have access to basic health and social care, regardless of availability); the rapid environmental changes and degradation of the environment; economic recession and crises in parts of the world that affect the financing of health care; the inability of technology to face epidemics and deadly threats from diseases such as HIV/AIDS, malaria, and tuberculosis; the growing crises and emergencies such as internal conflicts, civil wars, and natural disasters that affect the health delivery systems and access to care.

International health nurses are committed to care for all persons across the life cycle—pregnant women, infants, children, adolescents, adults, and the elderly—and especially vulnerable groups—the poor, refugees and displaced persons, street children, and the homeless.

In setting the future directions for global health policy, nursing and midwifery are key elements. As nurses and midwives already constitute up to 80% of the qualified health workforce in most national health systems, they represent a potentially powerful force for bringing about the necessary changes to meet the needs of health for all in the 21st century. Their contribution to health services covers the whole spectrum of health care, promotion and prevention, as well as health research, planning, implementation, and innovation.

EDUCATIONAL REQUIREMENTS

RN preparation is required; graduate preparation in nursing or public health is desirable.

CORE COMPETENCIES/SKILLS NEEDED

- Knowledge of major global health risks such as HIV/AIDS, tuberculosis, smoking, and environmental hazards
- Knowledge of epidemiology
- Skills in community mobilization for integrated health development
- Immunization knowledge and skills
- Leadership skills
- Skills in preparing nurses to be ready for emergencies and crisis situations

- Disaster planning and intervention skills
- Ability to enhance team building and leadership abilities of nurses as health care providers and planners
- Public health knowledge
- Skill in demonstrating cost-effective care through primary health care and the critical role of nurses in the health care team

RELATED WEBSITES AND PROFESSIONAL ORGANIZATIONS
- International Council of Nurses (www.icn.ch/index.html)
- Transcultural Nursing Society (www.tcns.org)
- World Health Organization (www.who.int)

INTERVENTIONAL RADIOLOGY NURSE

BASIC DESCRIPTION
The interventional radiology nurse is a professional nurse who cares for patients prior to, during, and following a procedure in interventional radiology. The nurse provides patient education, assesses patient needs, anticipates outcomes and side effects of procedures, and coordinates care and carrying out the plan of care.

EDUCATIONAL REQUIREMENTS
RN preparation is required. A bachelor's degree in nursing is preferred.

CORE COMPETENCIES/SKILLS NEEDED
- Excellent communication skills
- Thorough knowledge of interventional radiology procedures, protocols, and side effects/risks
- Ability to educate patients and families
- Ability to assist in necessary procedures

RELATED WEBSITE AND PROFESSIONAL ORGANIZATION
- Association for Radiologic & Imaging Nursing (www.arinursing.org)

145 INTERVENTIONAL RADIOLOGY NURSE PRACTITIONER

BASIC DESCRIPTION
The interventional radiology nurse practitioner—a practice role—works in either acute care settings or ambulatory centers caring for the patient undergoing radiologic imaging procedures and radiation oncology treatments. He or she is responsible for obtaining consents for the procedure, conducting a thorough physical assessment and medical–surgical history, and evaluating patients pre- and postprocedure.

EDUCATIONAL REQUIREMENTS
RN preparation, nurse practitioner certification, and basic life support and advanced cardiac life support certifications are required. A master's degree in nursing and several years of acute care experience as an RN, preferably in critical care or emergency nursing, are requirements.

CORE COMPETENCIES/SKILLS NEEDED
- Excellent assessment and critical thinking skills
- Excellent technical skills, such as placement of peripheral and central venous catheters and thoracotomy catheters
- Excellent organizational, leadership, and communication skills

RELATED WEBSITES AND PROFESSIONAL ORGANIZATIONS
- Association for Radiologic & Imaging Nursing (arinursing.org)
- Society of Interventional Radiology (www.scvir.org)

BASIC DESCRIPTION

Nurse inventors are those who seek solutions to patient care problems or delivery system problems by creating new devices; often these inventions are patented.

EDUCATIONAL REQUIREMENTS

RN preparation is required.

CORE COMPETENCIES/SKILLS NEEDED

- Desire to fix a problem that has arisen
- Desire to improve patient and nursing care
- Creativity
- Risk-taking skills
- Tenacity
- Innovativeness
- Belief in their product

RELATED WEBSITE AND PROFESSIONAL ORGANIZATION

- United States Patent and Trademark Office (www.uspto.gov)

147 IN VITRO FERTILIZATION NURSE

BASIC DESCRIPTION
Acting as coaches, guides, and support, in vitro fertilization (IVF) nurses assist patients in streamlining the processes involved in IVF. They coordinate diagnostic and treatment schedules and educate patients and their partners about medication administration, testing preparation, and specimen collection.

EDUCATIONAL REQUIREMENTS
RN preparation is required.

CORE COMPETENCIES/SKILLS NEEDED
- Knowledge of Food and Drug Administration regulations regarding fertility treatments
- Excellent organizational and communication skills
- Knowledge of diagnostic procedures and treatments and latest evidence-based information related to fertility and fertility treatment

RELATED WEBSITES AND PROFESSIONAL ORGANIZATIONS
- Resolve: The National Infertility Association (www.resolve.org)
- Society for Assisted Reproductive Technologies (www.sart.org)
- Society for Reproductive Endocrinology and Infertility (www.socrei.org)

JOINT COMMISSION CONSULTANT 148

BASIC DESCRIPTION
A consultant with The Joint Commission (TJC) provides consultation services to hospitals and health care organizations regarding organizational compliance with regulatory standards of TJC. TJC consultants provide on-site education and assistance to improve patient care in accordance with regulations. In this role, they are responsible for knowing up-to-date standards of TJC.

EDUCATIONAL REQUIREMENTS
RN preparation or other health care professional preparation is required, with a background in quality improvement. A minimum of a master's degree in a health care–related field is also needed.

CORE COMPETENCIES/SKILLS NEEDED
- Ability to travel 100% of the time
- In-depth knowledge of TJC standards and survey process
- Experienced leadership skills
- Ability to be direct
- Excellent oral and written communication skills
- Expert in quality assurance
- Current knowledge of health care issues and strategies
- Computer literacy
- Attention to detail and ability to be focused

RELATED WEBSITE AND PROFESSIONAL ORGANIZATION
- The Joint Commission (www.jointcommission.org)

149 LABOR AND DELIVERY NURSE

BASIC DESCRIPTION
A labor and delivery nurse works with mothers during the final stages of pregnancy helping with birthing, monitoring the mother's vital signs, and becoming astute in signs and symptoms of possible complications. These nurses are involved in patient education and addressing the psychosocial needs of mothers after delivery.

EDUCATIONAL REQUIREMENTS
RN preparation is required.

CORE COMPETENCIES/SKILLS NEEDED
- Excellent interpersonal and communication skills
- Excellent assessment skills to assess progression of labor
- Ability to provide support for the mother after childbirth and monitor the newborn immediately after birth

RELATED WEBSITES AND PROFESSIONAL ORGANIZATIONS
- American Nurses Credentialing Center (www.nursecredentialing.org/NurseSpecialties/Perinatal.aspx)
- Association of Women's Health, Obstetric and Neonatal Nurses (www.awhonn.org/awhonn)
- Perinatal Nursing Institute (perinatalnursingfw.org/wordpress)

LABOR AND DELIVERY NURSE ANESTHETIST

BASIC DESCRIPTION
A labor and delivery nurse anesthetist works with mothers during childbirth to minimize and/or relieve pain. The labor and delivery nurse anesthetist is expert at providing pain relief that is safe for both the mother and the baby. Further, the labor and delivery nurse anesthetist educates family members about different types of pain management strategies and assists them to choose the best pain relief strategy and anesthesia during labor.

EDUCATIONAL REQUIREMENTS
RN preparation and certification as a certified registered nurse anesthetist are required. Experience in labor and delivery as an RN is mostly required. Certification is offered by the National Board of Certification & Recertification of Nurse Anesthetists.

CORE COMPETENCIES/SKILLS NEEDED
- Sensitivity to the needs of the family
- Advanced knowledge of obstetrics
- Excellent communication skills in dealing with members of the obstetrics team

RELATED WEBSITES AND PROFESSIONAL ORGANIZATIONS
- American Association of Nurse Anesthetists (www.aana.com)
- International Federation of Nurse Anesthetists (ifna-int.org/ifna/news.php)
- National Board of Certification & Recertification of Nurse Anesthetists (www.nbcrna.com)

151 | LACTATION CONSULTANT NURSE PRACTITIONER

BASIC DESCRIPTION
A lactation consultant is an advanced practice nurse who assists expectant and post-partum mothers with breastfeeding and maintenance of newborn nutrition. Lactation consultants communicate with mothers to assess adequacy of breast milk production and newborn growth patterns. They are able to assist in breastfeeding techniques, prescribe medications or recommend supplements to enhance breast milk production, and provide guidance for issues related to breastfeeding. Furthermore, as a nurse practitioner, they can also assess, diagnose, and treat mothers and newborns for medical issues as needed during consultations.

EDUCATIONAL REQUIREMENTS
RN preparation is required. A Master of Science in Nursing with advanced practice certification as a nurse practitioner is required. Certification is available through the American Association of Colleges of Nursing and the American Nurses Credentialing Center. Basic life support and advanced cardiac life support certifications are also necessary. Certification as a lactation consultant is recommended.

CORE COMPETENCIES/SKILLS NEEDED
- Excellent communication, interpersonal, and teaching skills
- Thorough knowledge of physiology of lactation
- Knowledge of treatments and techniques to increase breast milk production
- Knowledge of normal growth and development of newborns

RELATED WEBSITES AND PROFESSIONAL ORGANIZATIONS
- American Association of Colleges of Nursing (www.aacn.nche.edu)
- American Nurses Credentialing Center (www.nursecredentialing.org)

LACTATION COUNSELOR

152

BASIC DESCRIPTION
Lactation and breastfeeding counselors work closely together when a mother experiences a breastfeeding problem. They assess the mother and baby, take her history, observe the mother and baby while breastfeeding, problem solve, develop a plan of care, work with and report to the mother's and baby's primary care providers, and arrange for follow-up.

EDUCATIONAL REQUIREMENTS
A lactation or breastfeeding counselor refers to anyone who is working in the field of lactation, either as a volunteer or as a professional. However, certification to become an International Board Certified Lactation Consultant is considered the gold standard. This exam is held once a year worldwide. Criteria that must be met for certification are bachelor's, master's, or doctoral degree—or 4 years of postsecondary education; a minimum of 2,500 hours of practice as a breastfeeding consultant; and a minimum of education specific to breastfeeding within the 3 years prior to the exam.

CORE COMPETENCIES/SKILLS NEEDED
- Excellent interpersonal skills
- Peer-counseling skills
- Excellent knowledge of lactation and women's health

RELATED WEBSITES AND PROFESSIONAL ORGANIZATIONS
- International Board of Lactation Consultant Examiners (www.iblce.org)
- International Lactation Consultant Association (www.ilca.org)
- La Leche League International (www.lalecheleague.org)

153 LEARNING/DEVELOPMENTAL DISABILITIES NURSE

BASIC DESCRIPTION
The role of a developmental disabilities nurse is to assist a client with mental and physical disabilities to live as normal and productive a life as possible. This might mean assisting clients with manual and recognition skills to enable them to carry out tasks related to maintaining activities of daily living, or developing comprehensive plans with specific goals and objectives. Developmental disabilities nurses work in sheltered workshops, group homes, long-term care facilities, and schools.

EDUCATIONAL REQUIREMENTS
RN preparation is required. Certification eligibility is available to RNs with a minimum of 4,000 hours (2 years full-time equivalent) of developmental disabilities nursing practice within the past 5 years.

CORE COMPETENCIES/SKILLS NEEDED
- Compassion and complete understanding of the person with a disability
- Patience
- Excellent communication skills
- Understanding of chronic long-term disabilities
- Counseling skills for families
- Ability to work with interdisciplinary teams
- Ability to promote positive life experiences
- Ability to provide care for health and social needs
- Ability to understand physical disabilities and psychological/emotional needs
- Ability to promote positive images of people with disabilities
- Ability to apply clinical and behavioral nursing interventions to meet the special health care needs of the individual
- Ability to act in the capacity of advocate
- Ability to maximize the client's potential by referring to appropriate resources
- Ability to manage care by coordinating services

RELATED WEBSITE AND PROFESSIONAL ORGANIZATION
- Developmental Disabilities Nurses Association (www.ddna.org)

BASIC DESCRIPTION
Legal nurse consultants (LNCs) are RNs who use specialized health care knowledge and expertise to consult on medical-related cases. Legal consultants provide a variety of services to attorneys, insurance companies, and hospitals in legal matters where health, illness, or injury are issues, such as personal injury, product liability, medical negligence, toxic torts, workers' compensation, risk management, and fraud and abuse. LNCs assist claims managers with the investigation, evaluation, and management of general and professional liability claims by obtaining, organizing, reviewing, and summarizing pertinent records and documents. They assist in the procurement of expert reviews and evaluation of care, and they provide input into the claims resolution strategy based on evaluations. They support managers with implementation of risk-management activities, all with the objective of controlling or minimizing losses to protect the assets of the corporation. Other responsibilities include drafting litigation documents, conducting medical and legal research, analyzing medical records in depth, and assisting the claims manager with investigation of general and professional liability claims. Employment opportunities are available in law firms, hospitals, insurance companies, governmental agencies, and consulting firms, as well as in the form of self-employment.

EDUCATIONAL REQUIREMENTS
RN preparation is required. Certification is available from the American Legal Nurse Consultant Certification Board.

CORE COMPETENCIES/SKILLS NEEDED
- Clinical experience, preferably in a high-risk area
- Statistical background/data management experience preferred
- Liability claims/paralegal experience, or educational equivalent also preferred
- Ability to work independently
- Ability to be a self-starter
- Confidence making decisions
- Excellent reading and writing skills
- Confidence to talk with experts

RELATED WEBSITES AND PROFESSIONAL ORGANIZATIONS
- American Association of Legal Nurse Consultants (www.aalnc.org)
- American Association of Nurse Attorneys (www.taana.org)
- Medical-Legal Consulting Institute, Inc. (www.legalnurse.com)

155 LEGISLATOR

BASIC DESCRIPTION

A nurse legislator is a nurse who is elected to public office. Nurse politicians serve in a variety of settings such as U.S. Congress, state government, boards of education, and nursing organizations. Given that there are more than 2.4 million nurses in this country, and that one in every 17 female voters is a nurse, this represents an important growth area for nursing influence. According to the American Nurses Association, the women currently serving in Congress who are nurses are Karen Bass from California's 33rd district, Diane Black from Tennessee's 6th district, Lois Capps from California's 24th district, Renee Elmer from North Carolina's 2nd district, and Eddie Bernice Johnson from Texas's 30th district.

EDUCATIONAL REQUIREMENTS

RN preparation is required. Education and/or experience in the area of political action is also necessary.

CORE COMPETENCIES/SKILLS NEEDED

- Conviction to fight for one's beliefs
- Interest in political and social issues
- Ability to be a decision maker
- Leadership ability
- Ability to identify a problem and develop a position and a plan to address the problem
- Ability to identify and articulate health care issues
- Skills in advocating for change
- Ability to collaborate with other members of the political team
- Knowledge to design legislation
- Experience in working for reforms in health care, education, and other identified areas of need

RELATED WEBSITES AND PROFESSIONAL ORGANIZATIONS

- American Nurses Association (www.ana.org)
- U.S. Congress (www.congress.gov)

BASIC DESCRIPTION

Life coaches are trained professionals who take their learned skills in health care and use them to help promote success, self-care, and wellness in their clients. They focus on counseling their clients by promoting an optimal level of health in the physical, spiritual, social, environmental, mental, emotional, professional, financial, and medical arenas. They use a variety of modalities to help people achieve a healthy lifestyle in a personalized way. They can also help people reach other goals in life outside of health care through motivation and resource management. A life coach can focus on coaching patients or helping other health care providers. Many nurses who become life coaches are entrepreneurs, but employment may also be found in educational or health care institutions.

EDUCATION REQUIREMENTS

Preparation as a registered nurse is not required, but is helpful. A degree in nursing, psychology, or another health care–related field is preferable. Certification is encouraged and is available through the International Association of Coaching and the International Coach Federation.

CORE COMPETENCIES/SKILLS NEEDED

- High level of motivation and ability to motivate others
- Creativity
- Ability to communicate effectively
- Self-awareness, perceptiveness, and intuition
- Ability to customize and personalize plans for clients
- Strong organizational skills
- Excellent interpersonal skills
- Knowledge of health and wellness techniques
- Strong coaching and educational skills
- Positive thinker
- Ability to inspire others and help them reach their health and life goals

RELATED WEBSITES AND PROFESSIONAL ORGANIZATIONS

- International Association of Coaching (www.certifiedcoach.org)
- International Association of Coaching Institutes (www.coaching-institutes .net)

- International Association of Professional Life Coaches (www .iaplifecoaches.org)
- International Coach Federation (www.coachfederation.org)
- International Coaching Association (www.internationalcoachingassociation .com)

LOBBYIST

BASIC DESCRIPTION
A nurse lobbyist is an advocate for nursing and other health care professions. Through the art of persuasion, sound legislative knowledge, excellent communication skills, and networking, they are able to influence legislative decisions that impact the practice of nursing. Large nursing organizations hire either a full-time lobbyist or a part-time consultant to advance their agenda.

EDUCATIONAL REQUIREMENTS
RN preparation is required. A master's degree is highly preferred.

CORE COMPETENCIES/SKILLS NEEDED
- Knowledge of state and federal laws that affect health care and political and legislative procedures
- Knowledge of the U.S. health care system
- Flexibility, professionalism, and excellent verbal and written communication skills

RELATED WEBSITES AND PROFESSIONAL ORGANIZATIONS
- American Nurses Association RN Action (www.rnaction.org/site/PageServer?pagename=nstat_homepage&ct=1)
- State Nurses Association

158 LONG-TERM CARE ADMINISTRATOR

BASIC DESCRIPTION

A long-term care administrator heads the overall management and operations of a long-term care facility. He or she oversees interdisciplinary departments in the facility that include nursing, medicine, rehabilitation, diet, activities, and environmental services, ensuring that resident and family needs, governmental and regulatory standards, and personnel needs are addressed while maintaining quality and excellent care. Nurses who have long-term care administrative and clinical experience and expertise are well positioned to assume this leadership role in long-term care facilities.

EDUCATIONAL REQUIREMENTS

A master's degree or higher in nursing, health, or business is preferred. Licensing and credentialing are available from the National Association of Long Term Care Administrator Boards. Certification is available from the National Association of Directors of Nursing Administration in Long Term Care.

CORE COMPETENCIES/SKILLS NEEDED

- Strong leadership and management skills
- Knowledge of state and federal regulations and the reimbursement process for long-term care
- Strong background in Medicare, Medicaid, and third-payer reimbursement regulations

RELATED WEBSITES AND PROFESSIONAL ORGANIZATIONS

- National Association of Directors of Nursing Administration in Long Term Care (www.nadona.org)
- National Association of Long Term Care Administrator Boards (www.nabweb.org/nabweb/default.aspx)

LONG-TERM CARE NURSE

BASIC DESCRIPTION

The long-term care nurse works in a long-term care facility with patients who have chronic physical and/or mental disorders, who are primarily elderly. Responsible for the day-to-day care of patients, operation of the facility, staff supervision, assessing program quality, program growth and development, and service excellence often are responsibilities of the long-term care nurse. Working in long-term care requires working with patients who have challenging diagnoses. Practice settings include nursing homes and skilled nursing facilities.

EDUCATIONAL REQUIREMENTS

RN preparation is required. Certification as gerontology nurse is available from the American Nurses Credentialing Center.

CORE COMPETENCIES/SKILLS NEEDED

- Prior experience with long-term care
- Medical and surgical nursing experience
- Ability to see death as a part of the natural process of life
- Ability to build long-term relationships with patients and their families
- Ability to build teams and mentor others
- Leadership and organizational ability
- Ability to solve staffing difficulties when they arise

RELATED WEBSITES AND PROFESSIONAL ORGANIZATIONS

- American Nurses Credentialing Center (www.nursecredentialing.org)
- Association for Long Term Care Nursing (aginginmotion.org/members/american-association-for-long-term-care-nursing)

MACROBIOTIC NUTRITIONIST

BASIC DESCRIPTION

A macrobiotic nutritionist is one who uses a diet plan based on whole grains, vegetables, and beans with the goal of helping clients achieve a more balanced and healthier lifestyle. Through coaching and planning, the macrobiotic nutritionist teaches his or her clients to eat regularly, listen to their bodies, stay active, chew adequately, and maintain mental positivity. These practices coupled with a pescatarian, low-fat, and high-fiber diet are thought to reduce the risk of illnesses. The professional background of a nurse can bring another dimension of holistic health approach to diet management.

EDUCATIONAL REQUIREMENTS

A bachelor's degree in clinical nutrition, dietetics, or a related field is required. A competency exam must be passed and registered dietician (RD) or registered dietician nutritionist (RDN) credential must be achieved. State licensing is required.

CORE COMPETENCIES/SKILLS NEEDED

- Excellent interpersonal skills
- Creativity with diets, food options, and recipes
- Skills in patient education
- Solid base of knowledge of macrobiotic diets

RELATED WEBSITES AND PROFESSIONAL ORGANIZATIONS

- Academy of Nutrition and Dietetics (www.eatright.org)
- American Society for Parenteral and Enteral Nutrition (www.nutritioncare.org)
- Commission on Dietetic Registration (www.cdrnet.org)
- National Board of Nutrition Support Certification by the American Society for Parenteral and Enteral Nutrition (www.nutritioncertify.org)

MAGNET® ACCREDITATION CONSULTANT

161

BASIC DESCRIPTION

A Magnet accreditation consultant is a nursing leader who is an expert in helping hospitals on their journey to Magnet designation or redesignation by the American Nurses Credentialing Center. This person works closely with nursing leadership at the institution to set a timeline with goals for application completion, conduct gap analysis, ensure that application requirements are met, that the document for submission is complete and sound, that the institution is well prepared for the on-site survey, and provide direction to institutions in need of improvement. Consultants can also host workshops to share knowledge of the application process to assist with submission. They can work independently or as part of a company.

EDUCATIONAL REQUIREMENTS

RN preparation is required. A minimum of a master's degree in nursing, health care administration, or a related field is necessary.

CORE COMPETENCIES/SKILLS NEEDED

- Critical thinking skills
- Thorough knowledge of Magnet application process and standards
- Ability to be highly organized
- In-depth understanding of standards of practice for nursing
- Strong interpersonal skills
- Excellent writing and oral communication skills
- Active listening skills
- Proficiency with computer programs
- Ability to work collaboratively and independently
- Excellent teaching or coaching skills
- Strong judgment skills
- Ability to analyze and synthesize information effectively and efficiently

RELATED WEBSITE AND PROFESSIONAL ORGANIZATION

- American Nurses Credentialing Center (www.nursecredentialing.org)

162 MAGNET® PROGRAM DIRECTOR

BASIC DESCRIPTION
Magnet program directors (or Magnet project coordinators) are nurse leaders who are responsible for leading their hospital on the journey to Magnet designation or redesignation. They collaborate and coordinate with various leaders within the hospital to collect data and information for application submission, educate nurses and nursing leadership on expectations and requirements for designation, prepare the nursing staff for the on-site survey, and instill excitement in the hospital regarding this process. They are ultimately responsible for completion and submission of the application document. In addition, the Magnet program director ensures that Magnet standards are integrated into the care delivery model that nurses integrate into their practice every day.

EDUCATIONAL REQUIREMENTS
RN preparation is required. A minimum of a master's degree in nursing, health care administration, or a related field is necessary.

CORE COMPETENCIES/SKILLS NEEDED
- Critical thinking skills
- Thorough knowledge of Magnet application process and standards
- Ability to be highly organized
- In-depth understanding of standards of practice for nursing
- Strong interpersonal skills
- Excellent writing and oral communication skills
- Active listening skills
- Proficiency with computer programs
- Ability to work collaboratively and independently
- Excellent teaching or coaching skills
- Strong judgment skills
- Ability to analyze and synthesize information effectively and efficiently
- Enthusiasm and passion for Magnet application process

RELATED WEBSITE AND PROFESSIONAL ORGANIZATION
- American Nurses Credentialing Center (www.nursecredentialing.org)

MAGNETIC RESONANCE IMAGING NURSE

163

BASIC DESCRIPTION
An MRI nurse works to provide nursing care specifically to patients, and often their families, who are undergoing an MRI procedure. An MRI is an imaging procedure that uses magnetic energy instead of radiation to view an organ or a body part. He or she can oversee staff in an MRI unit/suite, and work in a variety of patient care settings that can include inpatient services or ambulatory care services, and deal with all types of patient populations from children to older adults.

EDUCATIONAL REQUIREMENTS
RN preparation and basic life support certification are required. Certification as a radiology nurse is available.

CORE COMPETENCIES/SKILLS NEEDED
- Knowledge of care of patients specifically undergoing an MRI procedure
- Strong organizational, managerial, and leadership skills
- Excellent communication and interpersonal skills
- Strong assessment and critical thinking skills
- Computer literacy

RELATED WEBSITES AND PROFESSIONAL ORGANIZATIONS
- Association for Radiologic and Imaging Nursing (arinursing.org)
- *Journal of Radiology Nursing* (www.radiologynursing.org)
- Radiologic Society of North America (www.rsna.org)

164 MASSAGE THERAPY NURSE

BASIC DESCRIPTION
As a specialty, a massage therapist nurse uses a variety of touch therapies and other holistic approaches to facilitate a client's ability for self-healing.

EDUCATIONAL REQUIREMENTS
RN preparation with postgraduate education and 500 hours of training in massage and body therapies certified by the National Certification Board for Therapeutic Massage & Bodywork (NCBTMB).

CORE COMPETENCIES/SKILLS NEEDED
- Excellent communication skills
- Ability to adhere to NCBTMB code of ethics and standards of practice
- Knowledge of anatomy, physiology, kinesiology, pathology, professional standards, ethics, business, and legal practices

RELATED WEBSITES AND PROFESSIONAL ORGANIZATIONS
- American Massage Therapy Association (www.amtamassage.org/index.html)
- National Association of Nurse Massage Therapists (www.nanmt.org)
- National Certification Board for Therapeutic Massage & Bodywork (www.ncbtmb.org)
- United States Medical Massage Association (www.americanmedicalmassage.com)

BASIC DESCRIPTION

Nurses who are media consultants provide behind-the-scenes and upfront consultation for media in order to present accurate and realistic portrayals of health care, patient care, and the professional practice of nursing.

EDUCATIONAL REQUIREMENTS

RN preparation, but often RNs with advanced degrees and certifications in their specialty fields are preferred.

CORE COMPETENCIES/SKILLS NEEDED

- Knowledge of television, movie, and stage environments
- Ability to work with a wide variety of individuals from producers to actors
- Ability to work with deadlines
- Ability to work in a fast-paced, rapidly changing environment

RELATED WEBSITE AND PROFESSIONAL ORGANIZATION

- Registered Nurse Experts, Inc. (www.rnexperts.com)

166 MEDICAL CODING EDUCATOR

BASIC DESCRIPTION
A medical coding educator is responsible for providing training and education regarding up-to-date billing and coding processes, and information related to medical insurance and reimbursement to health care institutions. Included in this is developing an educational curriculum, identifying and meeting learning objectives, and providing educational resources. This person may also be involved in chart audits and quality assurance reviews to assess compliance and comprehension of this information by designated staff. He or she is responsible for ensuring continuing knowledge with updates in coding information.

EDUCATION REQUIREMENTS
Basic preparation or a degree in nursing, health information technology, or another health care–related field is required. A bachelor's degree is highly preferred. Experience with auditing and/or medical coding is also necessary. Certification is available and encouraged through the American Academy of Professional Coders.

CORE COMPETENCIES/SKILLS NEEDED
- Extensive knowledge of professional services medical coding
- Ability to be detail oriented
- Ability to thoroughly audit charts to evaluate compliance and quality performance
- Advanced knowledge of medical terminology, pharmacology, anatomy and physiology, and pathophysiology
- Excellent teaching and communication skills
- Proficiency in computer applications and electronic medical records
- In-depth knowledge of International Classification of Diseases (ICD)-9 and ICD-10, Current Procedural Terminology, and Healthcare Common Procedure Coding System guidelines
- Ability to analyze, interpret, and present statistics related to audits performed
- Ability to ensure compliance with organizational and regulatory standards
- Ability to create and execute effective learning curriculums

RELATED WEBSITE AND PROFESSIONAL ORGANIZATION
- American Academy of Professional Coders (www.AAPC.org)

MEDICAL DEVICE INVENTOR

BASIC DESCRIPTION
A medical device inventor works with medical device companies to design and manufacture new products. The company may provide funding, market review, device design and production, testing, proof of concept, market introduction and distribution, and ongoing management and support. The inventor can obtain a patent, license, or trademark for the product or device independently or through a company.

EDUCATION REQUIREMENTS
A bachelor's degree in nursing or a health care–related field is usually necessary. An educational background in engineering or business is also preferable. A master's degree is desirable in any of these fields as well.

CORE COMPETENCIES/SKILLS NEEDED
- Creativity and innovativeness
- Self-motivation
- Knowledge of the health care system and existing technologies and products
- Ability to collaborate with a team and to work independently
- Ability to be detail oriented and focused
- Persistence and goal orientedness
- Willingness to take risks
- Resilience and ability to recover from failure
- Passion about the project
- Ability to seek and create opportunities

RELATED WEBSITES AND PROFESSIONAL ORGANIZATIONS
- United States Patent and Trademark Office (www.uspto.gov)
- www.healthcareinventions.com

BASIC DESCRIPTION

A patient-centered medical home is a health care delivery model that uses a team-based approach to provide holistic and continuous care for patients in order to meet health care objectives. A medical home coordinator is a medical professional who coordinates care for clients using this model. He or she ensures timely, well-organized health care through multidisciplinary support services. Responsibilities include creation of care plans, referrals to community resources, scheduling of appointments, development of goals of care, follow-up after physician visits, communication and education, and helping patients solve other health care–related problems. This person can also be involved in performance improvement and quality assurance initiatives for the residents.

EDUCATIONAL REQUIREMENTS

A bachelor's degree in a health care–related field, such as nursing, is required. In some cases, an associate degree with significant health care field experience will be considered adequate.

CORE COMPETENCIES/SKILLS NEEDED

- Excellent writing and verbal communication skills
- Ability to collaborate and work as a team
- Excellent problem-solving and critical thinking skills
- Proficiency in computer programs
- Leadership and management skills
- Ability to be highly organized
- Cultural competence
- Superior customer service skills
- Ability to collect and analyze data
- Knowledge and ability to navigate health care system

RELATED WEBSITES AND PROFESSIONAL ORGANIZATIONS

There are no related websites or organizations.

MEDICAL RECORDS AUDITOR

169

BASIC DESCRIPTION
A medical records auditor examines, verifies, adjusts, and corrects medical records and bills to ensure accuracy and consistency. Medical records auditors report discrepancies to personnel and ensure corrective action is taken in a timely manner. They audit physician billing practices against documentation in the medical record to ensure compliance with all federal, state, and third-party billing requirements, rules, and regulations. They go through medical records to make sure everything is in compliance and all the codes match up for billing purposes.

EDUCATIONAL REQUIREMENTS
RN preparation is required. Many facilities also prefer that the applicant has some college-level business courses or health care experience.

CORE COMPETENCIES/SKILLS NEEDED
- Strong analytical skills and some basic training skills to teach people how to correct problems
- Basic knowledge of diagnostic-related groups and coding
- Broad knowledge of disease processes, findings, courses of treatment, quality assurance, and risk management

RELATED WEBSITES AND PROFESSIONAL ORGANIZATIONS
- Agency for Healthcare Research and Quality (www.ahrq.gov)
- National Association for Healthcare Quality (www.nahq.org)
- National Committee for Quality Assurance (www.ncqa.org)

170 MEDICAL–SURGICAL NURSE

BASIC DESCRIPTION
Medical–surgical nurses are RNs who specialize in the care of patients admitted with nonsurgical (medical) and surgical conditions. These nurses work to promote health, prevent disease, and help patients cope with illness. They are advocates and health educators for patients, families, and communities. The medical–surgical nurse has an incredibly complex job. The entry-level medical–surgical nurse makes nursing judgments based on scientific knowledge and relies on procedures and standardized care plans. Nursing care is directed toward alleviating physical and psychosocial health problems. Advancing to an intermediate level, the medical–surgical nurse with experience becomes more skilled in developing individual and innovative care plans to meet client needs. With a broader base of experience, a more advanced clinician cares for clients with complex and unpredictable problems. The most common place of employment is the hospital.

EDUCATIONAL REQUIREMENTS
RN preparation and, often, Master of Science in Nursing preparation are required. Certification is available through the American Nurses Credentialing Center and from the Academy of Medical–Surgical Nurses.

CORE COMPETENCIES/SKILLS NEEDED
- Excellent observation and assessment skills
- Skills in recording symptoms, reactions, and progress
- Skills in administering medical treatments and examinations
- Knowledge of convalescence and rehabilitation requirements for patients
- Skills in developing, planning, implementing, evaluating, documenting, and managing nursing care
- Patient and family education skills
- Ability to help individuals and groups take steps to improve or maintain their health

RELATED WEBSITES AND PROFESSIONAL ORGANIZATIONS
- Academy of Medical–Surgical Nurses (www.amsn.org)
- American Nurses Credentialing Center (www.nursecredentialing.org)
- Medical–Surgical Nursing Certification Board (msncb.org)

MILITARY NURSE

BASIC DESCRIPTION
Military nurses are those who serve in the military—army, navy, and air force in active duty, reserve, and civilian positions. Military nurses are among the most respected professionals in their field and enjoy many job-related benefits such as sign-on bonuses, housing allowances, and education loan repayment.

EDUCATIONAL REQUIREMENTS
RNs who have Bachelor of Science in Nursing degrees enter as officers; experience in acute care, such as critical care or emergency nursing, are desired qualities.

CORE COMPETENCIES/SKILLS NEEDED
- U.S. citizenship
- Must meet medical and moral standards outlined by the military
- Must pass a background security check
- Excellent communication skills
- Flexibility and ability to quickly adjust to different locations if deployed

RELATED WEBSITES AND PROFESSIONAL ORGANIZATIONS
- How to Become a Military Nurse (www.nmaetc.org/nursing/how-to-become-a-military-nurse)
- Information About Military Nursing (www.military-nurse.com)

172 MINDFULNESS COACH

BASIC DESCRIPTION
Mindfulness is a therapeutic practice of being consciously aware in the present moment of one's feelings, thoughts, and senses without passing judgment. A mindfulness coach uses techniques to help groups or individuals to increase or achieve mindfulness in order to improve perspective, reduce stress, promote wellness and self-development, and reach their potential. With a special set of skills from clinical knowledge and health care field experiences, a nurse is uniquely positioned to offer expertise as a mindfulness coach. A mindfulness coach can work independently hosting classes or personalized coaching sessions, or partner with a hospital, health care provider, or other health care agency to coach employees and patients.

EDUCATIONAL REQUIREMENTS
There is no specific educational requirement to be a mindfulness coach. However, one must be trained adequately in mindfulness and teaching mindfulness through various available modalities. For nurses, certification is available as a nurse coach through the International Nurse Coach Association.

CORE COMPETENCIES/SKILLS NEEDED
- Extensive knowledge about mindfulness and the practice of mindfulness
- Excellent people skills and ability to connect with people
- Nonjudgmental and compassionate
- Ability to be present
- Excellent teaching and coaching skills
- Reflectiveness and open mindedness
- Skills to deal with issues presented by the client
- Attentiveness

RELATED WEBSITE AND PROFESSIONAL ORGANIZATION
- International Nurse Coach Association (www.inursecoach.com)

BASIC DESCRIPTION

Minimum data set (MDS) nurses are long-term care nurses specializing in assessing the needs of long-term care residents. They are responsible for ensuring that MDS assessments are conducted regularly and that care is coordinated among long-term care residents. MDS is a tool that assesses quality of care among long-term care residents and that has a significant influence in payment and reimbursement of skilled nursing care provided.

EDUCATIONAL REQUIREMENTS

A Bachelor of Science in Nursing is often required; certification can be obtained from the American Association of Nurse Assessment Coordinators.

CORE COMPETENCIES/SKILLS NEEDED

- Ability to pay meticulous attention to details
- Knowledge of state and federal long-term care regulatory standards
- Basic computer skills
- Ability to work with interdisciplinary teams
- Significant long-term care experience

RELATED WEBSITE AND PROFESSIONAL ORGANIZATION

- American Association of Nurse Assessment Coordinators (www.aanac.org)

174 MISSIONARY NURSE

BASIC DESCRIPTION
Missionary nurses consider nursing as a calling and they provide nursing and spiritual care to those less fortunate and who may not share their religious belief or orientation. Some belong to a specific religious organization, and they usually work overseas. They assume various roles such as direct caregivers, nursing educators, nursing home administrators, and ambulatory care center directors.

EDUCATIONAL REQUIREMENTS
RN preparation is required.

CORE COMPETENCIES/SKILLS NEEDED
- Sensitivity to the needs of the less fortunate
- Ability to work and live overseas for an extended period
- Ability to speak other languages
- Strong interpersonal and communication skills
- Excellent clinical skills

RELATED WEBSITE AND PROFESSIONAL ORGANIZATION
- Discover Nursing (www.discovernursing.com/specialty/missionary-nurse#.V6Rh2vy_LGc)

MOTHER–BABY NURSE

BASIC DESCRIPTION
Mother–baby nurses provide holistic care to mothers and babies that includes patient education in areas of breastfeeding, diapering and bathing, umbilical cord care, and other safety areas in infant care. The mother–baby nurse also offers emotional support to mothers and their families, which is needed for a successful transition to parenthood. They must also be well versed in dealing with neonatal and maternal emergency situations.

EDUCATIONAL REQUIREMENTS
RN preparation is required; Bachelor of Science in Nursing is highly preferred; any experience in maternity or labor and delivery is highly desirable.

CORE COMPETENCIES/SKILLS NEEDED
- Knowledge of obstetrics, childbearing, and neonatal nursing
- Excellent teaching and communication skills
- Ability to work with members of health care team
- Strong computer and documentation skills
- Strong assessment and analytical skills

RELATED WEBSITE AND PROFESSIONAL ORGANIZATION
- Association of Women's Health, Obstetric and Neonatal Nurses (www.awhonn.org)

176 MOTIVATIONAL SPEAKER

BASIC DESCRIPTION
Nurses who function as motivational speakers are leaders in the field who desire to share knowledge, experience, perspective, or personal stories with nursing professionals around the world in order to inspire, empower, and inform their professional colleagues. Speakers can lecture on a wide array of topics, including stress management and reduction, teamwork, patient outcomes, health promotion, mindfulness, professional issues, professional development, and much more. Typically, speakers are self-employed and are hired to work at professional conferences, national observances, nurses' week celebrations, or at nursing appreciation events.

EDUCATION REQUIREMENTS
RN preparation is required. A bachelor's degree or master's degree in nursing is preferable. Experience and expertise in related field is necessary.

CORE COMPETENCIES/SKILLS NEEDED
- Expert knowledge in topic(s) of interest for lectures
- Ability to engage and motivate large audiences
- Self-motivation and self-promotion
- Excellent pubic speaking and communication skills
- Ability to travel
- Passion about topic of lecture
- High level of self-confidence
- Marketing skills

RELATED WEBSITE AND PROFESSIONAL ORGANIZATION
- www.speakersfornurses.com

BASIC DESCRIPTION

A nurse with a passion for writing novels can channel his or her nursing knowledge to become a mystery writer. In this role, a nurse can develop fictional novels or series based on real clinical scenarios or information with protagonists who are nurses. The possibilities are endless, and exciting storylines can be developed using nursing knowledge to contribute to the plotline. Most writers are freelancers; and many maintain a full-time job through an employer while writing.

EDUCATIONAL REQUIREMENTS

There is no educational requirement to become a writer. However, to write nursing-based novels, one must be prepared as an RN. A degree in English or creative writing is also advantageous.

CORE COMPETENCIES/SKILLS NEEDED

- Creativity
- Expert-level writing skills
- Patience
- Ability to work independently and meet deadlines
- Focus and self-motivation
- Passion for reading and writing
- Ability to accept criticism
- Health care–related knowledge

RELATED WEBSITES AND PROFESSIONAL ORGANIZATIONS

- Association of Authors' Representatives, Inc. (www.aaronline.org)
- Mystery Writers of America (http://mysterywriters.org)
- The Authors Guild (www.authorsguild.org)

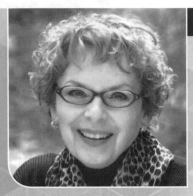

1. What is your educational background in nursing (and other areas) and what formal credentials do you hold?

I am a nurse author with experience both in nursing and in writing. Following several clinical and teaching positions, I became an associate dean and then a dean of nursing, as well as president of the nursing honor society, Sigma Theta Tau International. My credentials include an Associate Degree in Nursing, Bachelor of Science in Nursing, specializing in psychiatric nursing, and Doctor of Philosophy, and, more recently, coursework in creative writing.

2. How did you first become interested in your current career?

I wrote my first nursing book, *Effective Leadership and Management in Nursing*, because few nursing management books included content from organizational and management literature. That book is soon to be released in its ninth edition. Several other nursing books followed, including *Becoming Influential: A Guide for Nurses*, now in its second edition.

Like most nurses, I cringed at the inaccurate portrayal of nurses in books, movies, and television. As an avid reader of mysteries, I thought it might be fun to create a story using a nurse sleuth and depict nursing realistically. With my writing background, I thought I could transfer my skills to another genre. I couldn't have been more wrong!

After taking writing courses and attending workshops, and with the help of a talented (and ruthless) editor, my first mystery, *Twice Dead,* featuring nurse sleuth Monika Everhardt was published. Two more books in the series followed, *Deadly Diversion* and *Assumed Dead*. The last two were bought by Harlequin for their mystery line and are now e-books (see www .EleanorSullivan.com).

Continued

The success of the nursing mysteries inspired me to try historical fiction based on my family's ancestry. Set in a strict, religious society in 1830s rural Ohio, the stories feature a young midwife in a role anticipating nursing's future. Two books, *Cover Her Body* and *Graven Images*, have been published and a third, *Tree of Heaven*, will be released next year.

Today, the town in which I set these stories—Zoar, Ohio—is filled with museums, shops, and craftspeople demonstrating life in the 19th century. In 2017, the town will celebrate its bicentennial and, because of my books, I have been asked to write a play to commemorate the event. So, I am embarking on a completely new adventure in writing! *The Case of Goesele v. Bimeler* will tell the tale of the real-life trial that nearly destroyed the town.

3. What are the most rewarding aspects of your career?

Readers' opinions matter most. When people who are not nurses tell me they learned about nursing through my fiction, I feel satisfied that I met my goal. Similarly, nurse readers say that what they learned in *Becoming Influential*, they had never been taught in nursing school. Also, I know that my writing will survive me. It is my legacy for the future.

4. What advice would you give to someone contemplating the same career path in nursing?

Read everything you can, especially in the genre that interests you. Attend writers' events, join writers' organizations, take writing classes, and write, write, write. Get feedback on your work from other writers who are more experienced than you.

Contrary to popular opinion, writing is hard work. Start small. Write a letter to the editor, comment online about a current news story or offer to review a book for a community publication. Try coauthoring a clinical article with other nurses in your field. There is only one way to attain success as a writer: persistence. Persistence in learning your craft, persistence in accepting criticism, and persistence in submitting your work to potential markets are all necessary attributes of the published author.

You'll know you're a writer when you receive your first rejection. It won't be your last. Authors who are published didn't let that stop them. Don't let it stop you.

178 NEONATAL NURSE

BASIC DESCRIPTION
Neonatal nurses care for full or preterm babies specifically during the first 28 days of life. Neonatal nurses work with healthy newborns, those who need special care, such as preterm babies, or neonates who need constant monitoring and are critically ill.

EDUCATIONAL REQUIREMENTS
RN preparation is required; experience with pediatrics is highly preferred but not required. Pediatric advanced life support and neonatal advanced life support certifications are required in most positions. The National Certification Corporation offers certification in several neonatal nursing concentrations, and the American Association of Critical-Care Nurses offers certification in neonatal critical care nursing.

CORE COMPETENCIES/SKILLS NEEDED
- Knowledge of special and unique needs of the neonates and pediatric clients
- Excellent interpersonal and communication skills in working with families
- Excellent organizational skills
- Good grasp of math to accurately administer medications
- Excellent assessment and critical thinking skills

RELATED WEBSITES AND PROFESSIONAL ORGANIZATIONS
- Academy of Neonatal Nursing (www.academyonline.org)
- American Association of Critical-Care Nurses (www.aacn.org)
- Association of Women's Health, Obstetric and Neonatal Nurses (www.awhonn.org)
- National Association of Neonatal Nurses (www.nann.org)
- National Certification Corporation (www.nccwebsite.org/Certification/default.aspx)

NEONATAL NURSE PRACTITIONER

BASIC DESCRIPTION
Neonatal nurse practitioners (NNPs) are advanced practice nurses who specialize in providing care to acutely ill babies in the neonatal intensive care unit (NICU). These nurses have advanced skills in physical and psychosocial assessment of the newborn, and handle transport of acutely ill babies. The environments in which neonatal nurse practitioners work are very intense and dramatic, often with nonstop action.

EDUCATIONAL REQUIREMENTS
RN preparation and a Master of Science in Nursing with advanced practice certification as an NNP are required. Programs are generally of 2 years' duration. These programs are affiliated with major medical centers that are equipped to care for premature babies. Previous experience in the NICU is usually a requirement for admission to an NNP program.

CORE COMPETENCIES/SKILLS NEEDED
- Technical competency involving use of complex and computerized equipment
- Skill in regulating ventilators
- Hemodynamic monitoring skills
- Experience and expertise in assessing and managing acutely ill babies
- Skill in obtaining blood samples from central intravenous lines
- Interpersonal competency dealing with patients and their families in life-threatening situations
- Ability to work with interdisciplinary teams
- Ability to support parents' decisions even when you do not agree
- Comfort working with very small babies

RELATED WEBSITES AND PROFESSIONAL ORGANIZATIONS
- American Association of Nurse Practitioners (www.aanp.org)
- American Nurses Association Credentialing Center (www.ana.org)
- Association of Women's Health, Obstetric and Neonatal Nurses (www.awhonn.org)
- National Association of Neonatal Nurses (www.nann.org)

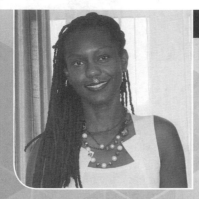

 PROFILE: MARIE B. FRANCOIS
Neonatal Nurse Practitioner

1. What is your educational background in nursing (and other areas) and what formal credentials do you hold?

I received an undergraduate degree from Princeton University, with a major in Spanish languages, then a Bachelor of Science in Nursing (BSN) via an accelerated program as a second undergraduate degree. I obtained a master's degree in nursing a few years later and am currently enrolled in a professional doctoral program (DNP). I am certified as an NNP. I have more than 10 years of nursing experience.

2. How did you first become interested in your current career?

Growing up, I had always been interested in the field of medicine. In college, premedicine was not a major so I took prerequisites such as organic chemistry and majored in Spanish languages in order to travel and expand my horizons. During my travels, a friend introduced me to the nurse practitioner career path. After graduating from college, I enrolled in an accelerated program to obtain my BSN and started working as a nurse in the NICU. The NICU is my first love in nursing care. The patients are tiny, fragile, and communicate nonverbally. I have worked in the NICU my entire career. While working as an RN, I continued my schooling and obtained my master's degree. I obtained my certification and started working as an NNP. I have now been enjoying this work for over 6 years. I find the work both challenging and fulfilling. I am obtaining my DNP in order to help incorporate the evidence found in research into our practice more efficiently as providers to these precious patients.

Continued

3. What are the most rewarding aspects of your career?

I enjoy working as part of a team to provide excellent care to our patients, and the respect garnered from members of our team. As I gain experience and seniority in my current position, I enjoy being able to share my knowledge with our fellows, residents, students, and new NNPs. Most importantly, I enjoy the flexibility that is offered by nursing and my position. I am able to travel extensively, and have a balance with my professional life and family.

4. What advice would you give to someone contemplating the same career path in nursing?

I would say "welcome to the profession." Nursing is awesome! You can do what you love, help people, garner respect, and still choose the lifestyle you want. There will be many people who ask, "Why didn't you become a physician?" My answer is that nursing is more holistic than medicine; nurses take care of the entire person, the whole family, and not just the illness. I love nursing because it encourages empathy. Nursing requires science as well as humanity. I would advise new nurses to always ask questions, never stop learning, and open themselves up to learning from all around them throughout their careers—including patients and their families.

180 NEPHROLOGY NURSE

BASIC DESCRIPTION
A nephrology nurse works with patients who have acute or chronic renal failure. He or she works with patients in all stages of renal disease and administers treatment, such as peritoneal dialysis and hemodialysis, in a variety of settings. Examples of places of employment include hospitals, outpatient clinics, dialysis settings, and patients' homes.

EDUCATIONAL REQUIREMENTS
RN preparation is required. Although not a requirement for employment, a certification in dialysis nursing is helpful. On-the-job training is a large part of becoming adept at dialysis nursing. It takes approximately 6 weeks to train a nurse with experience and about 6 months before nurses are truly comfortable and able to troubleshoot problems effectively.

CORE COMPETENCIES/SKILLS NEEDED
- Ability to assess even very subtle changes in the condition of a dialysis/nephrology patient
- Ability to understand and operate equipment used for hemodialysis
- Excellent interpersonal and communication skills, especially when working with patients and their families as they deal with chronic renal disease and its impact
- Ability to teach patients about renal disease, treatment, and lifestyle changes
- Ability to deal with grief and loss that can be associated with renal disease
- Collaboration and teamwork

RELATED WEBSITE AND PROFESSIONAL ORGANIZATION
- American Nephrology Nurses Association (www.annanurse.org)

NEPHROLOGY NURSE PRACTITIONER

181

BASIC DESCRIPTION
A nephrology nurse practitioner provides primary care to patients with acute or chronic kidney/urologic disorders, those undergoing dialysis, and those who are candidates for or have undergone kidney transplants.

EDUCATIONAL REQUIREMENTS
RN preparation and nurse practitioner certification are required. Certification is offered by the Nephrology Nursing Certification Commission.

CORE COMPETENCIES/SKILLS NEEDED
- Advanced knowledge in nephrology that includes pathophysiology and management of kidney/urologic conditions and their complications
- Excellent interpersonal, communication, and assessment skills
- Sensitivity to the needs of patients and their families as they deal with chronic renal disease and its impact
- Ability to teach patients about renal disease, treatment, and lifestyle changes
- Ability to deal with grief and loss that can be associated with renal disease
- Ability to work in a multidisciplinary team

RELATED WEBSITES AND PROFESSIONAL ORGANIZATIONS
- American Nephrology Nurses Association (www.annanurse.org/cgi-bin/WebObjects/ANNANurse.woa)
- Nephrology Nursing Certification Commission (www.nncc-exam.org/cgi-bin/WebObjects/NNCCMain)

182 NEUROLOGY/NEUROSCIENCE NURSE PRACTITIONER

BASIC DESCRIPTION

A neurology nurse practitioner is an advanced practice nurse who specializes in patient populations with neurological disease, spinal cord disease, brain and spinal cord injury, and stroke. Neurology nurse practitioners can work in critical care settings, such as a neurosurgical intensive care unit, inpatient neurology units, stroke services, private practice, community health centers, or outpatient neurological clinics. There are also positions for nurse practitioners to work in "cognitive fitness programs."

EDUCATIONAL REQUIREMENTS

RN preparation is required. Master of Science in Nursing with advanced practice certification as a nurse practitioner is required. Certification is available through the American Association of Nurse Practitioners and the American Nurses Credentialing Center. Basic life support and advanced cardiac life support certifications are also necessary.

CORE COMPETENCIES/SKILLS NEEDED

- Excellent assessment skills of brain and spinal cord functioning
- Ability to diagnose and treat neurological diseases
- Skill in patient and family education regarding condition and treatment options
- Skill in use of technology
- Extensive understanding of the nervous system, including anatomy and physiology, pathophysiology, medical treatments, and alternate therapies

RELATED WEBSITES AND PROFESSIONAL ORGANIZATIONS

- American Association of Neuroscience Nurses (www.aann.org)
- American Association of Nurse Practitioners (www.aanp.org)
- American Association of Spinal Cord Injury Nurses (www.aascin.org)
- American Nurses Credentialing Center (www.nursecredentialing.org)
- Brain Injury Association of America (www.biausa.org)
- World Federation of Neuroscience Nurses (www.wfnn.org)

NEUROLOGY NURSE

BASIC DESCRIPTION

A neurology nurse is one who cares for patients with acute stroke, traumatic brain injury, spinal cord injury, or other neurological diseases. Patients with neurological deficiencies require a special level of care and attention from nurses, as they are very complex patients who can be very dependent for activities of daily living. Neurology nurses work in inpatient settings on neurological units, home care agencies, neurosurgical intensive care units, or rehabilitation units.

EDUCATIONAL REQUIREMENTS

RN preparation is required. Basic life support is required. Certification as a Certified Neuroscience Registered Nurse is encouraged.

CORE COMPETENCIES/SKILLS NEEDED

- Skills in assessment of brain and spinal cord functioning
- Understanding of treatments for neurological diseases
- Skills in patient and family education
- Skills in use of technology
- Knowledge of the nervous system, including anatomy and physiology, pathophysiology, medical treatments, and alternate therapies

RELATED WEBSITES AND PROFESSIONAL ORGANIZATIONS

- American Association of Neuroscience Nurses (www.aann.org)
- American Association of Spinal Cord Injury Nurses (www.aascin.org)
- Brain Injury Association of America (www.biausa.org)
- World Federation of Neuroscience Nurses (www.wfnn.org)

184 NEUROSCIENCE NURSE

BASIC DESCRIPTION

Neuroscience nurses take care of individuals who have experienced changes in function or alterations in consciousness and cognition communication, mobility, rest and sleep, sensations, and sexuality. A nurse working in the neuroscience field should enjoy technology and working with people, and have both physical and psychological stamina.

EDUCATIONAL REQUIREMENTS

RN preparation is required. Certification is available from the American Board of Neuroscience Nursing.

CORE COMPETENCIES/SKILLS NEEDED

- Skills in patient and family education, especially regarding the neurological condition
- Skill in using the nursing process to plan and implement care
- Knowledge of neuroscience nursing, including anatomy and physiology, illness manifestations, and medical treatments
- Ability to manage families and individuals who are grieving loss
- Technological skills

RELATED WEBSITES AND PROFESSIONAL ORGANIZATIONS

- American Association of Neuroscience Nurses (www.aann.org)
- American Association of Spinal Cord Injury Nurses (www.aascin.org)

NURSE EXECUTIVE

BASIC DESCRIPTION

A nurse executive assumes a leadership role in a health care organization. He or she designs the institution's delivery of nursing care, plans and develops policies and procedures, assumes leadership in planning for the department's budget and fiscal needs, ensures adequate staffing, evaluates midlevel managers, and collaborates with other department heads.

EDUCATIONAL REQUIREMENTS

RN preparation and bachelor's degree, or higher, are required; certification is available from the American Nurses Credentialing Center.

CORE COMPETENCIES/SKILLS NEEDED

- Excellent leadership and management skills
- Strong communication and interpersonal skills
- Ability to work with members of other departments
- Knowledge related to budget and fiscal management
- Knowledge of leadership and management theories
- Knowledge and understanding of state and federal health care–related regulations
- Familiarity with Medicare, Medicaid, and third-party reimbursement
- Flexibility and ability to make quick decisions
- Objectivity, assertiveness, and excellent time management and organizational skills

RELATED WEBSITES AND PROFESSIONAL ORGANIZATIONS

- American Nurses Credentialing Center (www.nursecredentialingcenter.com)
- American Organization of Nurse Executives (www.aone.org)

186 NURSE MANAGER

BASIC DESCRIPTION

A nurse manager is responsible for the nursing care management of a certain patient care unit or a practice setting. A nurse manager has administrative and clinical responsibilities and mediates between staff and upper-level management. The employer outlines the nurse manager's responsibilities.

EDUCATIONAL REQUIREMENTS

RN preparation is required and a master's degree in nursing or management are highly preferred.

CORE COMPETENCIES/SKILLS NEEDED

- Excellent communication and interpersonal skills
- Advanced knowledge in the area of specialization
- Knowledge of leadership and management principles
- Knowledge of the organization's policies and quality improvement process
- Knowledge of state and federal accreditation guidelines
- Knowledge of budgeting and other fiscal matters

RELATED WEBSITES AND PROFESSIONAL ORGANIZATIONS

- American Organization of Nurse Executives (www.aone.org)
- Healthcare Performance Institute (www.healthcareperformanceinstitute.com)

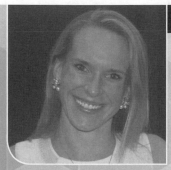

 PROFILE: LAURA STARK BAI

Clinical Nurse Manager,
Emergency Department (ED)

1. What is your educational background in nursing (and other areas) and what formal credentials do you hold?

I received a Bachelor of Science in Nursing and then, after 1 year of practicing clinically, I began a master's program with a family nurse practitioner focus. I am a board-certified family nurse practitioner. I am currently enrolled in a Doctorate of Nursing Practice program.

2. How did you first become interested in your current career?

My nursing career has been rather serendipitous. As a nursing student, I was placed in an ED for my senior practicum because my first choice (intensive care unit) was unavailable. During this time, I developed a passion for emergency nursing; therefore, I started my career as a nurse in the ED. After I completed my master's program, I was approached about a new leadership opportunity as the clinical nurse coordinator in my hospital's soon-to-be-opened ED observation unit. After accepting the position, I found that I enjoyed being in a leadership role, working to improve unit operations, the patient experience, and nursing quality. I then advanced to the position of clinical nurse manager of two new and innovative units in my hospital: the ED observation unit and the ED inpatient holding area. Now, I am happy to say that I have combined my passions for nursing leadership with emergency nursing, as I have just returned to the ED as clinical nurse manager.

3. What are the most rewarding aspects of your career?

I find many parts of my career to be rewarding. I have been able to be a part of the development and improvement of two innovative units. It has been exciting to learn more about inpatient nursing and observation nursing, and

Continued

PROFILE: LAURA STARK BAI
Continued

to help improve the operations of both units from their infancy. I am also continually gaining new knowledge and then sharing this knowledge with my staff to improve our practice and, therefore, patient outcomes. I am really looking forward to applying all that I have learned in the next step of my career as an ED nurse manager to contribute to the improvement and growth of the department. Finally, I love being a supportive resource to the nursing staff. I remember being a bedside nurse and looking up to and appreciating one of my unit's leaders, in particular because of her support and compassion, and I am honored to be able to serve my staff in the same way.

4. What advice would you give to someone contemplating the same career path in nursing?

The best advice I can give to nurses contemplating a career path in leadership is to never say "no." This applies to both the career and educational opportunities that one is exposed to, and to yourself and your goals. I have advanced to where I am in my career by taking advantage of all of the opportunities that have presented themselves to me and using them to grow in my role and expand my knowledge. I am constantly developing and building on skills that make me a better leader. The beautiful thing that I love about nursing is there are so many career options (as you can see in this book), and there is always more to learn that you can apply to your practice.

NURSE-MIDWIFE

187

BASIC DESCRIPTION
Certified nurse-midwives are advanced practice nurses who specialize in providing care to healthy women during pregnancy, childbirth, and after childbirth. Midwives provide accessible, safe birth care especially in rural and inner city areas. They teach patients and their families about the birthing process and provide the mother in labor birthing information and individualized attention. They provide care in a variety of settings including hospitals, birthing centers, clinics, homes, and offices.

EDUCATIONAL REQUIREMENTS
RN preparation plus a baccalaureate degree (not necessarily in nursing) are required to become a nurse-midwife. There are prerequisites that must be met but vary from one organization to another. The typical program averages 12 months, and a master's degree is the usual degree earned. The certification examination for nurse-midwives is offered through the American College of Nurse-Midwives Certification Council.

CORE COMPETENCIES/SKILLS NEEDED
- Strong assessment skills specifically related to this specialty
- Good communication ability
- Excellent leadership and organizational skills
- Understanding of relevant technology
- Ability to collaborate with other members of the health care team
- Compassion and caring attitude
- Ability to deal with a variety of people

RELATED WEBSITES AND PROFESSIONAL ORGANIZATIONS
- American College of Nurse-Midwives (www.acnm.org or www.midwife.org)
- American Midwifery Certification Board (www.amcbmidwife.org)
- Association of Women's Health, Obstetric and Neonatal Nurses (www.awhonn.org)

188 NURSE PSYCHOTHERAPIST

BASIC DESCRIPTION
Nurse psychotherapists work in a therapeutic relationship with their patients on either a one-to-one basis or in small therapy groups. Therapists form therapeutic alliances with their patients in order to help them to decrease their symptoms and to return to preillness level of function. Nurse psychotherapists work in a variety of settings including hospitals, clinics, and independent practice.

EDUCATIONAL REQUIREMENTS
RN preparation plus a master's degree and preparation as an advanced practice nurse are required. National certification by the American Nurses Credentialing Center in the specialty is required.

CORE COMPETENCIES/SKILLS NEEDED
- Advanced clinical skills in the area of psychiatric/mental health nursing
- Ability to practice independently in areas such as medication management and psychotherapy
- Ability to integrate research and theory into the practice of psychotherapy
- Ability to provide individual psychotherapy and psychiatric assessment
- Ability to integrate nursing science, computer science, and informatics in the provision of care
- Ability to work collaboratively with other specialty groups

RELATED WEBSITES AND PROFESSIONAL ORGANIZATIONS
- American Psychiatric Nurses Association (www.apna.org)
- Society for Education and Research in Psychiatric Mental Health Nursing (www.ispn-psych.org)

189

BASIC DESCRIPTION
A nursing home administrator is an individual who is responsible for overall functioning of a nursing home. This position involves managing and directing daily operations, making financial decisions, policy development and adherence, short- and long-term planning, and supervision of staff and residents to ensure optimal functioning and quality care for the nursing home residents.

EDUCATIONAL REQUIREMENTS
Educational and age requirements for nursing home administrators vary by state. A majority of states require a minimum of a bachelor's degree, but an associate degree may be acceptable. Licensure is required by successfully completing the exam through the National Association of Long Term Care Administrator Boards. Some states also require a state-based exam.

CORE COMPETENCIES/SKILLS NEEDED
- Excellent leadership and management skills
- Good computer skills
- Understanding of business
- Financial management skills
- Knowledge about aging process and effective care of the elderly
- Understanding of state and federal regulations and the reimbursement process
- Good interpersonal and communication skills

RELATED WEBSITES AND PROFESSIONAL ORGANIZATIONS
- National Association of Directors of Nursing Administration in Long Term Care (www.nadona.org)
- National Association of Long Term Care Administrator Boards (www.nabweb.org/nabweb/default.aspx)

190   NURSING SERVICES EDUCATOR

BASIC DESCRIPTION

A nursing services educator is a specialty nursing educator who focuses on the educational needs of nurses within a specific service line within a hospital or health system. Different service lines include, but are not limited to, medical, surgical, cardiac, emergency, psychiatric, pediatric, women's health, oncology, and perioperative. The service line educator assures that nurses' skills meet competency expectations for the institution, provides in-service training for new procedures or equipment, and provides just-in-time training and support for the nursing staff. They are also instrumental in orientation of the novice nurse or nurses new to an institution.

EDUCATIONAL REQUIREMENTS

RN preparation is required. A master's degree in nursing or education is highly preferred.

CORE COMPETENCIES/SKILLS NEEDED

- Strong interpersonal and communication skills
- Expertise in nursing skills and knowledge of service line
- Motivational, mentoring, and teaching skills
- Ability to manage multiple responsibilities
- Critical thinking and judgment skills
- Ability to remediate and offer constructive criticism
- Ability to nurture novice nursing staff
- Knowledge of institutional policies

RELATED WEBSITES AND PROFESSIONAL ORGANIZATIONS

- American Association of Colleges of Nursing (www.aacn.nche.edu)
- National League for Nursing (www.nln.org)

NURSING SPECIALTY COORDINATOR

BASIC DESCRIPTION

A nursing specialty coordinator is a nursing leader with comprehensive nursing knowledge and skills that work to coordinate patient care services and programs. The specialty coordinator works as an administrator with a specific patient population (e.g., cardiac patients, transplant patients, surgical patients) to promote interdisciplinary care, act as a resource for patients and families, manage quality indicators, and ensure patient satisfaction. In addition to patient services, the nursing specialty coordinator assesses and maintains nursing staff competency and acts as a resource for day-to-day operations of a nursing unit. Employment can be found in inpatient hospital settings or outpatient clinics.

EDUCATIONAL REQUIREMENTS

RN preparation is required. A minimum of a bachelor's degree in nursing is needed. A master's degree in nursing is preferred.

CORE COMPETENCIES/SKILLS NEEDED

- Strong clinical and interpersonal skills
- Assertiveness and excellent leadership skills
- Strong computer skills
- Ability to collaborate as part of a team
- Knowledge about nursing skills within specialty
- Critical thinking skills

RELATED WEBSITE AND PROFESSIONAL ORGANIZATION

- American Organization of Nurse Executives (www.aone.org)

192 NURSING SUPERVISOR

BASIC DESCRIPTION
The nursing supervisor oversees nursing and provides clinical leadership in a health care facility. He or she implements and interprets institutional policies and can also be involved in recruiting activities and preparing budgets.

EDUCATIONAL REQUIREMENTS
RN preparation is required. A Bachelor of Science in Nursing is required for most positions. Basic life support and advanced cardiac life support certifications, and at least 2 years' clinical experience are required.

CORE COMPETENCIES/SKILLS NEEDED
- Strong clinical and interpersonal skills
- Assertiveness and excellent leadership and managerial skills
- Knowledge of budgeting and accounting and leadership theories
- Strong computer skills and documentation skills
- Knowledge of collective bargaining agreement contracts
- Ability to work independently and make quick decisions
- Ability to work with other members of the health care team

RELATED WEBSITE AND PROFESSIONAL ORGANIZATION
- American Organization of Nurse Executives (www.aone.org)

NUTRITION ADVISOR

193

BASIC DESCRIPTION
A nutritionist is one who uses a diet plan to help clients achieve a more balanced and healthier lifestyle. Through coaching and teaching, the nutrition advisor teaches clients about how food choices affect their overall health. In this role, a nurse can use his or her unique set of skills and knowledge to help patients make optimal or necessary food and meal choices based on their medical needs, medical history, and medications that they take to promote health and wellness.

EDUCATIONAL REQUIREMENTS
A bachelor's degree in clinical nutrition, dietetics, or a related field is required. A competency exam must be passed and a registered dietician or registered diet nutritionist credential must be obtained. State licensing is also required.

CORE COMPETENCIES/SKILLS NEEDED
- Excellent interpersonal skills
- Creativity with diets, food options, and recipes
- Skill in patient teaching
- Ability to manage acute and chronic access devices
- Skill in guidelines and protocols on patient nutrition support

RELATED WEBSITES AND PROFESSIONAL ORGANIZATIONS
- Academy of Nutrition and Dietetics (www.eatright.org)
- American Society for Parenteral and Enteral Nutrition (www.nutritioncare.org)
- Commission on Dietetic Registration (www.cdrnet.org)
- National Board of Nutrition Support Certification by the American Society for Parenteral and Enteral Nutrition (www.nutritioncertify.org)

BASIC DESCRIPTION

Nutrition support nurses play a major role in the maintenance of patients' nutritional health. While most patients are able to eat or may just require some encouragement and assistance, some patients are unable to meet their nutritional needs via the oral route. The provision of nutrition support, which includes enteral feeding (via the gastrointestinal tract) and total parenteral nutrition (via the venous circulation), allows maintenance or repletion of the nutritional status for this group of patients. Nutrition support is provided by a multidisciplinary team comprising nurse clinicians, dieticians, gastroenterologists, surgeons, and pharmacists. The nurse clinician and team coordinate, provide, and advise patients on nutrition support. The team ensures that patients' nutritional needs are met by the safest, most economical, and most efficacious nutritional modality. Often the work includes assistance for children who require special nutritional intervention, including those with feeding disorders, growth failure, dietary intolerance, short bowel syndrome and congenital bowel disorders, and malabsorption. Nutrition support services can be provided to administer long-term intravenous nutrition or specialized tube feedings in selected cases.

EDUCATIONAL REQUIREMENTS

RN preparation is required. Certification is offered by the National Board of Nutrition Support Certification by the American Society for Parenteral and Enteral Nutrition.

CORE COMPETENCIES/SKILLS NEEDED

- Skill in developing guidelines and protocols on patient nutrition support
- Ability to manage the various acute and chronic nutritional access devices, both enteral as well as parenteral
- Skill in developing, implementing, and evaluating appropriate programs for staff training and patient teaching
- Interdisciplinary team skills
- Ability to work in a range of health care settings

RELATED WEBSITES AND PROFESSIONAL ORGANIZATIONS

- American Society for Parenteral and Enteral Nutrition (www.nutritioncare.org)
- National Board of Nutrition Support Certification by the American Society for Parenteral and Enteral Nutrition (www.nutritioncertify.org)

OBSERVATIONAL MEDICINE NURSE

BASIC DESCRIPTION

Observation units, also known as "clinical decision units," are a new branch of emergency departments that function to care for patients who do not meet inpatient admission criteria, but require ongoing observation, treatment, and/or testing. Nurses who work in observation units care for these patients for up to 48 hours. They work closely with an interdisciplinary team to provide care and facilitate disposition or discharge or admission.

EDUCATIONAL REQUIREMENTS

RN preparation is required. A minimum of an associate degree in nursing is needed; a bachelor's degree in nursing is preferred.

CORE COMPETENCIES/SKILLS NEEDED

- Ability to think critically and help expedite decision making
- Knowledge in treatment of a wide range of diagnoses
- Ability to work collaboratively with a team
- Efficient and able to keep up with a high turnover environment

RELATED WEBSITE AND PROFESSIONAL ORGANIZATION

- Emergency Nurses Association (www.ena.org)

196 OCCUPATIONAL HEALTH NURSE

BASIC DESCRIPTION
Occupational health nurses work in a variety of settings to keep workers healthy and to prevent work-related injuries. These nurses provide direct care services to employees on the job, host health-promotion activities, and provide workers' compensation case management. They are also often responsible for treatment of hazards in specific work environments. Practice settings include businesses, industries, government facilities, and shopping malls.

EDUCATIONAL REQUIREMENTS
RN preparation is required; a Bachelor of Science in Nursing is often preferred, and graduate education may be required. Usually 2 years of medical–surgical experience is required. Certification in specialized occupational health nursing roles is available from the American Board for Occupational Health Nurses, Inc.

CORE COMPETENCIES/SKILLS NEEDED
- Knowledge of Occupational Safety and Health Administration (OSHA) regulations and workers' compensation laws
- Ability to maintain, protect, and preserve the health of employees in their work environment
- Ability to analyze and prioritize risk factors to achieve highest level of health among employees
- Ability to coordinate care
- Assist in meeting OSHA standards
- Ability to provide health education
- Ability to manage crises/emergencies
- Autonomy
- Innovative thinking
- Good communication skills
- Excellent health assessment skills
- Effective managerial skills

RELATED WEBSITES AND PROFESSIONAL ORGANIZATIONS
- American Association of Occupational Health Nurses (www.aaohn.org)
- American Board for Occupational Health Nurses, Inc. (www.abohn.org)

OCCUPATIONAL HEALTH NURSE PRACTITIONER

BASIC DESCRIPTION

Occupational health nurse practitioners work with employees to ensure safe workplace conditions by conducting routine physical assessments, educating workers about hazard control, providing vaccinations, and counseling on health-promoting lifestyle. They make important recommendations to organizations that could lead to increased employee retention and job satisfaction.

EDUCATIONAL REQUIREMENTS

RN preparation, nurse practitioner certification, and basic life support certification are required; clinical experience as an RN in ambulatory or acute care settings is required. Certification is available from the American Board for Occupational Health Nurses.

CORE COMPETENCIES/SKILLS NEEDED

- Knowledge of workplace regulations such as those outlined by the Occupational Safety and Health Administration, Health Insurance Portability and Accountability Act, and the Family and Medical Leave Act
- Excellent interpersonal and communication skills
- Strong computer and documentation skills
- Strong organizational skills

RELATED WEBSITE AND PROFESSIONAL ORGANIZATION

- American Association of Occupational Health Nurses (www.aaohn.org)

198 OFFICE NURSE

BASIC DESCRIPTION
Office nurses perform routine administrative and clinical tasks to keep the offices and clinics of family practice physicians, internal medicine, oncologists, cardiologists, surgeons, advanced practice nurses, and others running smoothly. The goal of the office nurse is to provide personalized and efficient service to the patients they serve. They often play an important role in uncovering problems or concerns of the patient and alerting the physician of these issues. They perform telephone triage and provide patient education about many routine topics. They care for the patients in offices, clinics, surgical centers, and emergency medical centers. Depending on the type of facility, the office nurse serves patients with a variety of needs—diagnostic, medication, monitoring, wound treatment, maintenance, preventive medicine, surgery, and education. One of the most important responsibilities of an office nurse is telephone triage, integrating appropriate attention to biological and psychosocial issues with high-quality medical care. Another vital role for office nurses is that of patient advocate. Duties vary from office to office, depending on location, size, and specialty. Administrative duties often include answering telephones, greeting patients, updating and filing patient medical records, filling out insurance forms, handling correspondence, scheduling appointments, arranging for hospital admission and laboratory services, and handling billing and bookkeeping.

EDUCATIONAL REQUIREMENTS
RN preparation is required; experience is often a major requirement, but there are classes available to enhance telephone triage skills.

CORE COMPETENCIES/SKILLS NEEDED
- Good communication skills
- Knowledge of disease processes and normal development
- Office management skills
- History-taking and physical assessment skills
- Patient and family education
- Knowledge of medications
- Skill in routine nursing activities such as dressing changes, vital signs, and assessment

RELATED WEBSITE AND PROFESSIONAL ORGANIZATION
- American Academy of Ambulatory Nursing (www.aaacn.org)

OMBUDSMAN

BASIC DESCRIPTION

An ombudsman is someone who investigates reported complaints, reports findings, and helps achieve equitable settlements. He or she handles complaints and concerns regarding the quality of life and the quality of care of vulnerable adults receiving long-term care services. Activities performed include information and referral, problem solving, conflict resolution, mediation, and education. Because of the nature and diversity of the complaints and concerns, there is a need to work with many state and local organizations. The sources of the complaints are varied from the clients themselves, to their families, provider staff, doctors, representatives from state agencies, and hospital discharge planners. The complaints range from straightforward to multifaceted. For example, some need specialized equipment, and some have restraint concerns. Complaints may also include inadequate staffing, financial exploitation, alleged staff abuse, family conflicts, cold food, lost laundry, poor infection control, and decubitus ulcers. Ombudsmen work with the Department of Health, the regulatory agency for all health care facilities in the long-term care continuum. They are often closely involved with the departments of elderly affairs, human services, mental health and retardation, and hospitals, as they are providers and payers of care to the targeted population. They also work closely with the state's attorney general's office, attorneys, and the probate court system. As part of an organization, there is involvement in many committees, task forces, and councils, leading to legislative activities.

EDUCATIONAL REQUIREMENTS

RN preparation is required. Nursing background and experience are of benefit because of many concerns regarding clinical issues. It is also beneficial to have nursing input due to the high acuity levels of people receiving long-term care services along with the dealings with the hospitals, the medical community, and the nursing industry at all levels. Families and clients also feel added reassurance that a nurse is involved.

CORE COMPETENCIES/SKILLS NEEDED
- Excellent listening and interpersonal skills
- Skill in documentation
- Flexibility

- Ability to work with individuals from a variety of backgrounds
- Management skills required for dealing with a large number of agencies and representatives

RELATED WEBSITE AND PROFESSIONAL ORGANIZATION

- United States Ombudsman Association (www.usombudsman.org)

ONCOLOGY NURSE

BASIC DESCRIPTION
An oncology nurse cares for patients with cancer in various stages of the disease. Most patients experience problems from both the disease and the treatment. Oncology nurses administer chemotherapy, manage symptoms and the effects of treatment, and care for the needs of their patients with empathy. They must also deal with the psychological ramifications that the diagnosis of cancer brings as well as with the issues related to death and dying. Oncology nurses may be employed in a variety of settings. They most often work in special oncology units within hospitals, but may work in outpatient areas, home care, and hospice care.

EDUCATIONAL REQUIREMENTS
RN preparation is required; a Bachelor of Science in Nursing (BSN) or higher degree in nursing may be required. Some agencies may require certification as an oncology nurse.

CORE COMPETENCIES/SKILLS NEEDED
- Ability to cope with human suffering, emergencies, and other stresses
- Maturity
- Excellent interpersonal and communication skills
- Strong teaching ability
- Ability to adapt to new treatment regimens
- Knowledge of drugs used in chemotherapy
- Strong knowledge background in disease processes and symptom management in particular forms of cancer

RELATED WEBSITES AND PROFESSIONAL ORGANIZATIONS
- Association of Pediatric Hematology/Oncology Nurses (www.aphon.org)
- Oncology Nursing Certification Corporation (www.oncc.org)
- Oncology Nursing Society (www.ons.org)

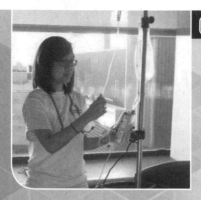

PROFILE: JILL SAN JUAN

Oncology Nurse

1. What is your educational background in nursing (and other areas) and what formal credentials do you hold?

I graduated in 2009 with a BSN. I am a registered nurse in Ohio and Texas. As a nurse working on an oncology floor (more specifically, a leukemia unit), I am also certified in administering chemotherapy and vesicants.

2. How did you first become interested in your current career?

In high school, community service hours were required for each year. I volunteered at a local hospital and was introduced to bedside interaction with patients. With oncology, I first became interested in the field during a summer externship of my junior year. I appreciated the technical and emotional aspects of the field. Oncology is fast paced and requires a high level of critical thinking. It is also an area where you build a special bond with your patients and families.

3. What are the most rewarding aspects of your career?

The most rewarding aspect of my oncology career is being by the patient and families from new diagnoses and throughout treatment. The continuity of care in oncology is unique because a typical hospital stay for a patient is a month (from being newly diagnosed and throughout whichever treatment he or she chooses). Staff members on the floor really invest themselves in the patients, get to know them very well, and can become their sole support system. It is extremely rewarding to see your patient come back and visit the staff on the unit just to thank them for all that they do. This has happened many times!

Continued

PROFILE: JILL SAN JUAN
Continued

4. **What advice would you give to someone contemplating the same career path in nursing?**

Nursing is an evolving career. Nursing is not limited to being in a hospital setting. A nurse can expand his or her role by teaching classes at nursing schools, to working at a village in South America. Nursing is an extremely rewarding career for you and your patients. It is an area for personal growth. There are always opportunities to advance in your career if you are ready for a change.

201 ONCOLOGY NURSE PRACTITIONER

BASIC DESCRIPTION
As primary care providers, oncology nurse practitioners (NPs) provide comprehensive care to patients who have a diagnosis of cancer, as well as to their families. In collaboration with health care team members, the oncology NP conducts a thorough physical assessment, writes prescriptions for medications, administers therapeutic measures, and evaluates care provided.

EDUCATIONAL REQUIREMENTS
RN preparation and NP certification are required. There are several certifications available for oncology NPs such as the advanced oncology certified nurse practitioner and advanced oncology certified nurse specialist by the Oncology Nursing Certification Corporation.

CORE COMPETENCIES/SKILLS NEEDED
- Excellent assessment, leadership, and critical thinking skills
- Ability to work with members of the health care team
- Excellent organizational and fiscal skills

RELATED WEBSITES AND PROFESSIONAL ORGANIZATIONS
- Oncology Nursing Certification Corporation (www.oncc.org/TakeTest/Certifications/AOCNP)
- Oncology Nursing Society (www.ons.org)

BASIC DESCRIPTION

Operating room nurses are RNs who perform direct patient care to patients undergoing surgery or other invasive procedures. They can be involved in the preoperative, operative, or postoperative stages of surgery. As a result, their role may function based on the phase of the process in which they work. For example, a scrub nurse or a circulating nurse will work inside of the operating room to fulfill their responsibilities. A postanesthesia care nurse, however, will deliver a high level of nursing care to a patient in the immediate period following the surgical procedure. Other responsibilities include assessing patients prior to surgery, monitoring the patient during surgery, maintaining a safe and sterile surgical environment, acting as a liaison between the surgical team and families during surgery, and teaching patients and families about postoperative care. Operating room nurses work closely with surgeons, anesthesiologists, nurse anesthetists, surgical technicians, and surgical assistants. Locations for employment include hospitals, ambulatory surgery centers, clinics, or private practice.

EDUCATIONAL REQUIREMENTS

RN preparation is required. Basic life support certification and often advanced cardiac life support certification are also required. Multiple certifications are available, including Certified Perioperative Nurse (CNOR), Certified RN First Assistant (CRNFA), and Certified Perioperative Clinical Nurse Specialist (CNS-CP). Certification is encouraged and can be obtained through the Competency and Credentialing Institute.

CORE COMPETENCIES/SKILLS NEEDED
- Ability to maintain levelheadedness in times of stress
- Collaboration skills
- Good communication skills
- Knowledge of the surgical process and the risks and benefits of surgical intervention
- Critical thinking skills
- Ability to stand for long periods of time
- Excellent assessment skills

RELATED WEBSITES AND PROFESSIONAL ORGANIZATIONS
- American Association of Critical-Care Nurses (www.aacn.org)
- Association of periOperative Registered Nurses (www.aorn.org)
- Competency and Credentialing Institute (www.cc-institute.org)

203 OPHTHALMIC NURSE

BASIC DESCRIPTION
An ophthalmic nurse cares for patients with disorders and diseases relating to the eyes. Ophthalmic nursing is full of opportunities for dedicated and highly skilled nurses who want to work with patients with ophthalmic diseases. Although it is a specialized field, it is also a career full of opportunities for nurses who want to use their general nursing knowledge and skills. Work settings include ophthalmologists' offices, hospitals, ambulatory surgery centers, research laboratories, and eye banks.

EDUCATIONAL REQUIREMENTS
RN preparation is required. The National Certifying Board for Ophthalmic Registered Nurses is an independently incorporated organization supported by the American Society of Ophthalmic Registered Nurses for the purpose of developing and implementing the certifying process for ophthalmic RNs. Candidates who meet the following criteria are eligible to take the certification examination for ophthalmic registered nurses: currently licensed as an RN in the United States or having the equivalent hours (4,000) of experience in ophthalmic RN practice; completion and filing of an application for certification examination for ophthalmic RNs.

CORE COMPETENCIES/SKILLS NEEDED
- Ability to provide psychosocial support for patients and families
- Excellent communication skills
- Understanding of diseases of the eye and treatment protocols
- Ability to work in the operating room to assist with operative procedures

RELATED WEBSITES AND PROFESSIONAL ORGANIZATIONS
- American Society of Ophthalmic Registered Nurses (www.asorn.org)
- National Certifying Board for Ophthalmic Registered Nurses (www.asorn.org)

ORGAN DONATION COUNSELOR

BASIC DESCRIPTION
An organ donation specialist/counselor is a nurse who works with families who have loved ones with irrevocable injuries and are on life support, and discusses the possibility of organ donation. There is a critical shortage of tissue and organ donation for transplants, and nurses can play a vital role in eliminating this shortage. Organ donation nurses are highly specialized and there are many related responsibilities. The education of nurses as designated requesters may have a considerable impact on the number of donors, because nurses are close to prospective donors and their families. Nurses provide a vital connection in the organ donation process.

EDUCATIONAL REQUIREMENTS
RN preparation is required. There are many programs that educate nurses to become donation requesters. The American Board of Transplant Coordinators offers two certifications to transplant coordinators after working in the field for a minimum of 1 year. Certification is available as either a certified procurement transplant coordinator or a certified clinical transplant coordinator.

CORE COMPETENCIES/SKILLS NEEDED
- Maturity
- Familiarity with types of donation and donation criteria
- Knowledge of the agency policy
- Knowledge of the types of transplantations
- Familiarity with different religious positions regarding tissue and organ donation
- Ability to deal with issues related to death and dying

RELATED WEBSITES AND PROFESSIONAL ORGANIZATIONS
- American Board for Transplant Certification (www.abtc.net/Pages/default .aspx)
- International Transplant Nurses Society (www.itns.org)
- North American Transplant Coordinators Organization (www.natco1.org)

205 ORTHOPEDIC NURSE

BASIC DESCRIPTION
Orthopedic nurses care for patients of all ages who have actual and potential musculoskeletal injuries and conditions. An orthopedic nurse may provide assessments and educate patients about braces, prosthetics, and other orthopedic equipment. The nurse must be interested in the care of patients before and after surgery involving the musculoskeletal system, such as total hip replacement, arthroscopy, total knee replacement, or spinal surgery. Orthopedic nursing is full of opportunities for dedicated and highly skilled nurses who want to work with patients with orthopedic conditions. Work settings include sports medicine clinics, sports franchises, hospitals, clinics, and ambulatory surgery centers.

EDUCATIONAL REQUIREMENTS
RN preparation is required. The Orthopaedic Nurses Certification Board provides a credentialing mechanism that validates proficiency in orthopedic nursing practice. Candidates who meet the following criteria are eligible to take the examination: currently licensed as an RN; 2 years of professional nursing practice; and having a minimum of 1,000 hours of work experience in orthopedic nursing within the past 3 years.

CORE COMPETENCIES/SKILLS NEEDED
- Excellent communication skills
- Understanding of the laws of physics
- Interest in sports and physical activity

RELATED WEBSITES AND PROFESSIONAL ORGANIZATIONS
- National Association of Orthopaedic Nurses (www.orthonurse.org)
- Orthopaedic Nurses Certification Board (www.oncb.org)

OTOLARYNGOLOGY NURSE

BASIC DESCRIPTION
An otolaryngology nurse focuses on care for patients with acute and chronic diseases relating to the head and neck. They assess and provide direct patient care to patients of all ages with disorders of the throat, ears, eyes, nose, skin, oral cavities, and cranial nerves. They also provide support for patients undergoing invasive procedures involving the head and neck. Work places include hospital, community health centers, outpatient private practices or clinics, and ambulatory care facilities.

EDUCATIONAL REQUIREMENTS
RN preparation is required. Basic life support certification is also required. Certification is encouraged and available through the Society of Otorhinolaryngology and Head-Neck Nurses.

CORE COMPETENCIES/SKILLS NEEDED
- Good assessment skills, especially of the head and neck
- Understanding of disorders affecting the head and neck, including treatment options
- Good communication and documentation skills
- Ability to provide emotional support

RELATED WEBSITES AND PROFESSIONAL ORGANIZATIONS
- American Head & Neck Society (www.ahns.info)
- Otorhinolaryngology Head & Neck Nurses Group Inc. (www.ohnng.com.au)
- Society for Ear, Nose and Throat Advances for Children (www.sentac.org)
- Society of Otorhinolaryngology and Head-Neck Nurses (www.sohnnurse.com)

207 PAIN MANAGEMENT NURSE

BASIC DESCRIPTION
The pain management nurse collaborates with an interdisciplinary team in the management of patients with acute and chronic pain. Pain management is a Joint Commission on Accreditation standard and is a critical need of many patients. Opportunities exist to work in acute care settings, outpatient clinics, rehabilitation centers, and home care.

EDUCATIONAL REQUIREMENTS
RN preparation is required. Certification in pain management is available from the American Nurses Credentialing Center and from the American Academy of Pain Management.

CORE COMPETENCIES/SKILLS NEEDED
- Empathy and understanding
- Understanding of the physiological and psychological aspects of pain
- Excellent communication skills
- Ability to work with interdisciplinary teams
- Interest in the complex issues regarding pain and the control of pain

RELATED WEBSITES AND PROFESSIONAL ORGANIZATIONS
- American Academy of Pain Management (www.aapainmanage.org)
- American Nurses Credentialing Center (www.nursecredentialing.org)
- American Society for Pain Management Nurses (www.aspmn.org)

PAIN MANAGEMENT NURSE PRACTITIONER

BASIC DESCRIPTION

A pain management nurse practitioner provides a holistic approach to assessing, diagnosing, and managing acute and chronic pain across all age groups in a variety of health care settings. The pain management nurse practitioner incorporates evidence-based approaches in implementing pharmacological and nonpharmacological interventions to alleviate pain and its associated symptoms.

EDUCATIONAL REQUIREMENTS

RN preparation, nurse practitioner certification, and basic life support certification are required.

CORE COMPETENCIES/SKILLS NEEDED

- Sensitivity in dealing with patients and families
- Knowledge of palliative nursing and end-of-life care
- Excellent interpersonal and communication skills
- Excellent assessment and analytical skills and ability to work with the pain management team
- Excellent clinical and technical skills such as phlebotomy and medication administration

RELATED WEBSITES AND PROFESSIONAL ORGANIZATIONS

- American Pain Society (www.ampainsoc.org)
- American Society for Pain Management Nursing (www.aspmn.org)

209 PALLIATIVE CARE NURSE PRACTITIONER

BASIC DESCRIPTION
A palliative care nurse practitioner provides comprehensive care to patients and families living with a terminal illness. They could develop practice protocols for end-of-life care, educate other clinicians about palliative care, conduct research to expand knowledge about palliative care, and assume administrative roles in health care organizations.

EDUCATIONAL REQUIREMENTS
RN preparation and nurse practitioner certification are required. Most positions require 1 year of acute care experience; certification is offered by the National Board for Certification of Hospice and Palliative Nurses.

CORE COMPETENCIES/SKILLS NEEDED
- Advanced knowledge and preparation in pain and symptom management and end-of-life care
- Sensitivity to the needs of terminally ill patients and their families
- Knowledge of hospice regulations and standards of care
- Excellent communication and assessment skills
- Strong computer and documentation skills
- Ability to work with an interdisciplinary team that includes physicians, social workers, dietitians, and unlicensed assistive personnel

RELATED WEBSITES AND PROFESSIONAL ORGANIZATIONS
- Center to Advance Palliative Care (www.capc.org)
- Hospice and Palliative Nurses Association (http://hpna.advancingexpertcare.org)
- National Board for Certification of Hospice and Palliative Nurses (www.nbchpn.org)

PARISH NURSE

BASIC DESCRIPTION

A parish nurse is a registered nurse who facilitates the holistic health of a congregation by focusing on spiritual, emotional, and physical dimensions of a person. Parish nurses act as a liaison and a facilitator in church, community, and hospital settings, and work with clergy in meeting the physical and spiritual needs of members of a particular congregation. Activities of parish nurses include community screenings (e.g., taking blood pressures, patient teaching, making home visits, counseling, and patient advocacy).

EDUCATIONAL REQUIREMENTS

RN preparation is required.

CORE COMPETENCIES/SKILLS NEEDED

- Interest in helping members of a congregation maintain optimum levels of health and independent living
- Excellent communication skills
- Ability to express care and compassion
- Strong religious affiliation
- Ability to provide patient and family education
- Excellent assessment skills
- Advocacy skills

RELATED WEBSITES AND PROFESSIONAL ORGANIZATIONS

- Faith Communities Partnering for Wellness (www.npnm.org/npnm_programs0.aspx)
- Health Ministries Association, Inc. (hmassoc.org)

211 PATIENT CARE COORDINATOR

BASIC DESCRIPTION
Patient care coordinators are responsible for ensuring that patients are receiving high quality medical care from a health care facility. They work closely with patients, families, an interdisciplinary health care team, and hospital administration to ensure care delivery goals are met. In addition, they work to implement patient care coordination initiatives, assist with case management, and work with administration to create and improve policies.

EDUCATIONAL REQUIREMENTS
An associate or bachelor's degree in a health care–related field is required. Often, RN preparation is required.

CORE COMPETENCIES/SKILLS NEEDED
- Excellent interpersonal skills
- Excellent communication skills
- Critical thinking and problem-solving skills
- Ability to navigate the health care system
- Knowledge of institutional policies
- Strong writing skills
- Ability to collaborate as a member of a team

RELATED WEBSITES AND PROFESSIONAL ORGANIZATIONS
There are no related websites or organizations.

PATIENT EDUCATION COORDINATOR

BASIC DESCRIPTION
The patient education coordinator is responsible for educating patients about their disease, medications, and all aspects of care needed following hospitalization or a clinic visit. Patient education is intended to help patients and families cope with a crisis, gather information, learn self-care, and use attitudes and strategies to promote optimal health. Patients who are well informed about their own health actively make their own health care decisions, are more likely to have better health overall and enjoy a better quality of life, have fewer illness-related complications, tend to be more compliant with medication and treatment regimens, and are less likely to be a drain on diminishing health care resources. Opportunities are available to work in hospitals, clinics, schools, health care organizations, and home health agencies.

EDUCATIONAL REQUIREMENTS
RN preparation with a Bachelor of Science in Nursing is required. A Master of Science in Nursing is preferred in most settings.

CORE COMPETENCIES/SKILLS NEEDED
- Ability to teach and inspire others
- Maturity and dependability
- Excellent communication skills
- Ability to work with interdisciplinary teams
- Knowledge about pathophysiology and health promotion
- Interest in teaching patients to manage acute and chronic illness
- Ability to plan health education programs
- Ability to prepare teaching materials
- Ability to develop patient teaching plans in a form that is readily understood by them and pertinent to their unique circumstances

RELATED WEBSITES AND PROFESSIONAL ORGANIZATIONS
- Health Care Education Association (www.hcea-info.org)
- National Council on Patient Information and Education (www.talkaboutrx.org)

213 PATIENT EXPERIENCE DIRECTOR

BASIC DESCRIPTION
The patient experience director is a leadership position for a nurse in which he or she works with executive leadership to ensure that goals related to patient satisfaction are being met within an organization. Patient experience directors are ultimately responsible for planning and implementing initiatives to improve the patient experience that are consistent with the institution's mission, vision, values, and care model. They also work closely with nursing leadership to identify areas for improvement for patient satisfaction and develop plans to achieve these identified goals. The patient experience director also works with a team that organizes and operates training programs to educate frontline providers on customer satisfaction and communication skills. Employment opportunities are generally in hospitals and health care systems.

EDUCATION REQUIREMENTS
RN preparation is required. However, training in another health care specialty is also accepted in some institutions. A bachelor's degree in nursing or a health care–related field is necessary. A master's preparation is highly preferred.

CORE COMPETENCIES/SKILLS NEEDED
- Outstanding customer satisfaction and interpersonal skills
- Ability to communicate effectively and compassionately
- Excellent leadership and management skills
- Ability to be highly organized
- Coaching and/or teaching skills
- Ability to analyze, interpret, and present data
- Proficiency in computer skills
- Expert knowledge on subject of patient experience
- Ability to manage challenging situations
- Critical thinking skills

RELATED WEBSITES AND PROFESSIONAL ORGANIZATIONS
- Association for Patient Experience (www.patient-experience.org)
- Hospital Consumer Assessment of Healthcare Providers and Systems (www.hcahpsonline.org)
- Press Ganey (www.pressganey.com)

PATIENT NAVIGATOR

BASIC DESCRIPTION

A patient navigator acts as a liaison who helps patients navigate the health care system to ensure timely, appropriate care. They assist patients in scheduling appointments, setting up appropriate referrals, accessing resources, and by answering questions to ensure understanding. Patient navigators can work as part of a hospital or in an outpatient setting.

EDUCATIONAL REQUIREMENTS

RN preparation or other health care training is required. A minimum of an associate's degree in a health care–related field is necessary.

CORE COMPETENCIES/SKILLS NEEDED

- Excellent communication skills
- Proficiency in computer programs
- Strong interpersonal skills and ability to advocate for patients
- Knowledge of how to navigate the health care system
- Critical thinking and problem-solving skills
- Ability to work in a fast-paced environment
- Ability to work as part of a team

RELATED WEBSITE AND PROFESSIONAL ORGANIZATION

- Patient Navigator Training Collaborative (www.patientnavigatortraining.org)

215

PATIENT REVIEW INSTRUMENT NURSE ASSESSOR

BASIC DESCRIPTION
This specialized long-term care nurse role is to assess the appropriateness of long-term care placement of patients. Assessment areas include the patient's physical, cognitive, and medical conditions. In some states, the patient review instrument (PRI) is used to determine skilled care needs of long-term care residents.

EDUCATIONAL REQUIREMENTS
RN preparation is required.

CORE COMPETENCIES/SKILLS NEEDED
- Knowledge of state and federal regulatory standards for long-term care
- Excellent organizational and assessment skills
- Ability to communicate with members of the health care team and patient's family or significant others
- Knowledge of the health care needs of older adults

RELATED WEBSITES AND PROFESSIONAL ORGANIZATIONS
- Hospital and Community Patient Review Instrument and Screen Training Certification Program (www.albany.edu/sph/cphce/pri-screen.shtml)
- Island Peer Review Organization (www.ipro.org)

PEACE CORPS VOLUNTEER

BASIC DESCRIPTION

Peace Corps volunteer nurses are assigned to specific jobs in developing countries. The history of the Peace Corps is the story of tens of thousands of people who have served as volunteers since 1961. Their individual experiences have comprised a legacy of service that has become part of American history. This is a 27-month commitment. These health volunteers work in both rural and urban settings where they raise awareness about the need for health education and infrastructures for healthy environments. They work on a variety of health activities in the community, from educating and training in the areas of maternal/child health, basic nutrition, sanitation, oral rehydration therapy, and sexually transmitted diseases/AIDS to organizing fund-raisers and community groups to obtain needed health care materials. Volunteers construct wells, tap springs, build latrines, improve potable water storage facilities, and train local leaders to maintain water and sanitation systems and continue health programs after the volunteers depart. They teach in classrooms and model methodologies for teachers in local schools and undertake knowledge, attitude, and practice surveys; assist clinics and/or ministerial planning offices in pinpointing health needs; devise educational projects to address prevailing health conditions; assist in the marketing of messages aimed at improving local health practices; and carry out epidemiological studies.

EDUCATIONAL REQUIREMENTS

RN preparation is required.

CORE COMPETENCIES/SKILLS NEEDED

- Flexibility
- Patience
- Maturity
- Curiosity
- Enthusiasm for helping people
- Dedication
- Compassion
- Understanding of different cultures
- Desire to make a difference in a developing country
- Excellent clinical skills

RELATED WEBSITE AND PROFESSIONAL ORGANIZATION

- Peace Corps (www.peacecorps.gov)

217 PEDIATRIC CARDIAC NURSE ANESTHETIST

BASIC DESCRIPTION
A pediatric cardiac nurse anesthetist is part of the pediatric cardiac anesthesia team responsible for the care of children undergoing cardiac surgery and other cardiovascular procedures, such as electrophysiologic studies. The pediatric cardiac nurse anesthetist is responsible for meeting the patient and the family before the operation to explain what to expect during and after the procedure.

EDUCATIONAL REQUIREMENTS
RN preparation and certification as a certified registered nurse anesthetist are required. Experience in acute or emergency care is mostly required. Basic life support, pediatric advanced life support, and advanced cardiac life support certifications are required; certification is offered by the National Board of Certification & Recertification of Nurse Anesthetists.

CORE COMPETENCIES/SKILLS NEEDED
- Ability to work with members of the team
- Excellent communication skills and sensitivity when addressing the needs and concerns of the family and the patient
- Excellent assessment skills and advanced knowledge in cardiovascular, pulmonary, and hemodynamic physiology, management, and pharmacology
- Ability to work in a high-stress environment that requires quick decisions in cases of emergency and sudden change in patients' hemodynamic status
- Ability to involve in light-to-moderate lifting as required with individual patient care

RELATED WEBSITES AND PROFESSIONAL ORGANIZATIONS
- American Association of Nurse Anesthetists (www.aana.com)
- International Federation of Nurse Anesthetists (ifna-int.org/ifna/news.php)
- National Board of Certification & Recertification of Nurse Anesthetists (www.nbcrna.com)

BASIC DESCRIPTION

A pediatric nurse is responsible for the nursing care of patients from infancy to late teens. They work in varied health care settings that range from ambulatory centers to acute care facilities. They may also work in specialized settings such as surgery, cardiology, rehabilitation, and oncology.

EDUCATIONAL REQUIREMENTS

RN preparation and basic life support certification are required. A thorough orientation is required for those who have no pediatric experience, especially among new graduates. Certification is offered either by the Pediatric Nursing Certification Board or by the American Nurses Credentialing Center after passing an exam and completing practice hours. The American Association of Critical-Care Nurses offers a certification in pediatric critical care nursing.

CORE COMPETENCIES/SKILLS NEEDED

- Flexibility in working with pediatric patients and their families
- Knowledge of unique needs of pediatric patients, including growth and development and common disease conditions

RELATED WEBSITES AND PROFESSIONAL ORGANIZATIONS

- American Nurses Credentialing Center (www.nursecredentialing.org)
- Pediatric Nursing Board Certification Board (www.pncb.org)
- Society of Pediatric Nurses (www.pedsnurses.org)

219 PEDIATRIC NURSE ANESTHETIST

BASIC DESCRIPTION

A pediatric nurse anesthetist cares for children during surgery or other medical or surgical procedures. He or she works in collaboration with anesthesiologists and could be employed in many settings, such as the operating room and ambulatory care centers. During the delivery of anesthesia, the pediatric nurse anesthetist monitors the patient's level of consciousness, body functions, and responses to the procedure and intervenes if there is a need. He or she works with the patient and families to make the hospital stay as pleasant as possible.

EDUCATIONAL REQUIREMENTS

RN preparation and certification as a certified registered nurse anesthetist are required. Experience as an RN in pediatrics is mostly required for most positions; certification is offered by the National Board of Certification & Recertification of Nurse Anesthetists.

CORE COMPETENCIES/SKILLS NEEDED

- Excellent communication skills
- Excellent assessment and analytical skills
- Advanced knowledge in pediatrics and sedation

RELATED WEBSITES AND PROFESSIONAL ORGANIZATIONS

- American Association of Nurse Anesthetists (www.aana.com)
- International Federation of Nurse Anesthetists (ifna-int.org/ifna/news.php)
- National Board on Certification & Recertification of Nurse Anesthetists (www.nbcrna.com)

PEDIATRIC NURSE PRACTITIONER

BASIC DESCRIPTION

Pediatric nurse practitioners are advanced practice nurses who provide management of care for acutely and/or chronically ill pediatric patients. Hospitalization is frightening for a child, so the pediatric nurse specialist must know how to alleviate or assist in alleviating fears of children and their families. Children of a young age are often unable to express their emotions; therefore, it is the responsibility of the pediatric nurse specialist to be alert to and aware of unexpressed needs. Work settings include acute care settings, subacute care settings, long-term care facilities, home care agencies, health maintenance organizations, ambulatory care settings, and schools.

EDUCATIONAL REQUIREMENTS

A Bachelor of Science in Nursing, advanced practice licensure, a Master of Science in Nursing in pediatrics or family health, and pediatric advanced life support certification are required. Continuing education for maintenance of licensure is also a requirement. Certification is available from the American Nurses Credentialing Center (ANCC). A certification as a pediatric clinical nurse specialist is also available from the ANCC.

CORE COMPETENCIES/SKILLS NEEDED
- Special knowledge of growth and development
- Knowledge of pediatric illnesses and their treatment
- Ability to function independently
- Ability to work with children and their families
- Ability to set priorities and work independently
- Ability to collaborate with other health care providers

RELATED WEBSITES AND PROFESSIONAL ORGANIZATIONS
- American Nurses Credentialing Center (www.nursecredentialing.org)
- Association of Pediatric Hematology/Oncology Nurses (www.aphon.org)
- National Association of Pediatric Nurse Practitioners (www.napnap.org)
- Pediatric Nursing Certification Board (www.pncb.org/ptistore/control/index)
- Society of Pediatric Nurses (www.pedsnurses.org)

221 PEDIATRIC ONCOLOGY NURSE

BASIC DESCRIPTION
The pediatric oncology nurse—a highly specialized and sensitive role—delivers care to those pediatric patients who are receiving cancer treatment. Specific responsibilities include preparing patients for chemotherapy, administering palliative treatment, and collaborating with other members of the health care team.

EDUCATIONAL REQUIREMENTS
RN preparation and basic life support certification are required. Pediatric advanced life support certification is required for most positions; certification is offered by the Oncology Nursing Certification Corporation.

CORE COMPETENCIES/SKILLS NEEDED
- Knowledge of pediatric oncology
- Knowledge of safe handling of chemotherapeutic drugs
- Excellent communication, interpersonal, and assessment skills
- Flexibility and sensitivity of the unique needs of the pediatric oncology patients

RELATED WEBSITES AND PROFESSIONAL ORGANIZATIONS
- Association of Pediatric Oncology Nurses (www.apon.org)
- Oncology Nursing Certification Corporation (www.oncc.org)
- Oncology Nursing Society (www.ons.org)

PERFORMANCE IMPROVEMENT DIRECTOR

BASIC DESCRIPTION

The director of performance improvement is responsible for the design, implementation, and evaluation of quality and performance improvement activities of a health care organization.

EDUCATIONAL REQUIREMENTS

RN preparation is required; a master's degree is required in most positions. Certification as a certified professional in health care quality is highly preferred.

CORE COMPETENCIES/SKILLS NEEDED

- Strong statistical skills
- Knowledge of federal and state health regulations, accreditation
- Knowledge of health policy, budget and fiscal-related matters, case management, risk management, and infection control
- Knowledge of grant-writing activities to fund initiatives
- Strong written and verbal communication skills

RELATED WEBSITES AND PROFESSIONAL ORGANIZATIONS

- Healthcare Quality Certification Board (www.cphq.org)
- National Committee on Quality Assurance (www.cphq.org)
- National Organization of Competency Assurance (www.noca.org)

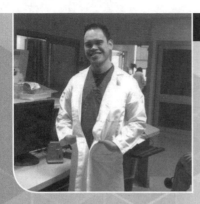

 PROFILE: **JASON TAN**

Performance Improvement Coordinator

1. What is your educational background in nursing (and other areas) and what formal credentials do you hold?

I have two bachelor's degrees, in business administration and in nursing, and an MBA in quality management.

2. How did you first become interested in your current career?

After finishing my first bachelor's degree, in business administration, I entered the corporate world. I was a stockbroker on Wall Street for a private firm. I then moved into banking. I left banking looking for something more meaningful. I wanted to be in a profession that would not only be gratifying but also something where I could grow as an individual professionally.

My mother, who has been an emergency room nurse for over 30 years, recommended that I consider a career in nursing. I originally was against it and had the stereotypical view that nursing was only for women. Through much research, volunteer work, and support of family and friends, I decided to go back to school to become a nurse.

3. What are the most rewarding aspects of your career?

It is rewarding to me to simply be able to help people day in and day out in their time of need. Every day brings a new challenge, and I can leave my job knowing I was able to advance the health of a patient. The gratification from the patients is a reward in itself.

Continued

4. **What advice would you give to someone contemplating the same career path in nursing?**

Try to expose yourself to the multiple areas in nursing. Find an area that you can be passionate about and truly love. Learn as much as you can and pursue the direction you want to go in with the understanding that you will be helping someone in their time of need.

223 PERIANESTHESIA NURSE

BASIC DESCRIPTION
Perianesthesia nursing provides intensive care to patients as they awake from anesthesia. Perianesthesia nurses prepare patients for the surgical experience, monitor and support safe transition from anesthetized state to responsiveness, and ready patients for discharge from the perianesthesia care unit. They have opportunities to work in perianesthesia care units in inpatient and outpatient settings, including freestanding operative settings, hospitals, and clinics.

EDUCATIONAL REQUIREMENTS
RN preparation is required. Certification is available. There are two certification programs for qualified registered nurses: the Certified Postanesthesia Nurse (CPAN) program and the Certified Ambulatory Perianesthesia Nurse (CAPN) program.

CORE COMPETENCIES/SKILLS NEEDED
- Experience in medical–surgical and critical care nursing
- Hands-on skills such as line placement, tube insertions, dressing changes, intravenous therapy, and positioning
- Flexibility
- Good assessment and decision-making skills
- Good management skills
- Technological abilities
- Ability to teach
- Good interpersonal skills
- Ability to respond to possible complications of anesthesia, including respiratory compromise, hypotension, emergence excitement, nausea and/or vomiting, and pain
- Flexibility and an ability to manage stress

RELATED WEBSITES AND PROFESSIONAL ORGANIZATIONS
- American Board of Perianesthesia Nursing Certification, Inc. (www.cpancapa.org)
- American Society of PeriAnesthesia Nurses (www.aspan.org)

PERINATAL NURSE 224

BASIC DESCRIPTION
A perinatal nurse cares for women, infants, and their families from the onset of pregnancy through the first month of the newborn's life (perinatal period). The perinatal nurse needs to convey to the provider the patient's physiological status (vital signs, contractions, physical examination findings) and the well-being of the fetus, as evidenced by fetal heart auscultation or monitoring, in clear language. Perinatal nurses have opportunities to work in hospitals including specialty hospitals, health departments, medical offices, health maintenance organizations, clinics, birthing centers, nurse-midwife practices, and home health agencies.

EDUCATIONAL REQUIREMENTS
RN preparation is required. Certification in perinatal nursing is available.

CORE COMPETENCIES/SKILLS NEEDED
- Interpersonal skills
- Commitment
- Oral and written communication skills
- Ability to monitor the pregnancy
- Ability to assess the progression of labor and maintain a sense of calm and comfort during labor
- Ability to monitor the status of mother and baby
- Knowledge of family support
- Skill in fostering the new mother–infant relationship and teaching parenting skills
- Ability to assess and support the mother in her recovery from childbirth as well as evaluate the newborn's early adjustment to life

RELATED WEBSITES AND PROFESSIONAL ORGANIZATIONS
- American Nurses Credentialing Center (www.nursingworld.org/ancc)
- Association of Women's Health, Obstetric and Neonatal Nurses (www.awhonn.org)
- National Association of Neonatal Nurses (www.nann.org)

225 PERIOPERATIVE NURSE

BASIC DESCRIPTION
A perioperative nurse is a member of a surgical team who provides care for a patient before, during, and immediately after the patient has experienced a surgical intervention.

EDUCATIONAL REQUIREMENTS
RN preparation is required. Certification is available through the Association of Operating Room Nurses or from the Competency and Credentialing Institute.

CORE COMPETENCIES/SKILLS NEEDED
- Knowledge and skills needed to assist in preparing and operating the technological tools involved in new surgical techniques now available (e.g., lighter fiberoptic scopes/lenses and video monitors)
- Skill in providing comfort to the patient
- Skill in assisting the anesthetic caregivers
- Respect for cultural diversity, patients' rights, privacy, and confidentiality
- Team skills for interactions with surgeons, surgical technologists, other nurses, anesthesiologists, nurse anesthetists, pathologists, radiologists, perfusionists, support assistant staff, and many other members of the health care team
- Skill in facilitating patient advocacy
- Excellent basic nursing skills in observation and assessment

RELATED WEBSITES AND PROFESSIONAL ORGANIZATIONS
- Association of periOperative Registered Nurses (www.aorn.org)
- Competency and Credentialing Institute (www.cc-institute.org)

PERIOPERATIVE NURSE PRACTITIONER 226

BASIC DESCRIPTION

The primary responsibility of a perioperative nurse practitioner is to conduct a thorough physical assessment of patients scheduled for an operative procedure, screen for potential complications during and after surgery, order preoperative laboratory tests and interpret their results, and provide patient teaching and anticipatory guidance.

EDUCATIONAL REQUIREMENTS

RN preparation and nurse practitioner certification are required. Basic life support certification is required, and advanced cardiac life support certification is preferred in most positions. Certification as adult nurse practitioner from the American Academy of Nurse Practitioners National Certification Program is available.

CORE COMPETENCIES/SKILLS NEEDED

- Excellent assessment and analytical skills
- Strong computer skills
- Ability to work in a fast-paced dynamic environment
- Ability to work in a team

RELATED WEBSITES AND PROFESSIONAL ORGANIZATIONS

- American Academy of Nurse Practitioners (www.aanp.org/AANPCMS2)
- Association of periOperative Registered Nurses (www.aorn.org)

227 PHARMACEUTICAL REPRESENTATIVE

BASIC DESCRIPTION
The pharmaceutical representative is an RN involved in promoting and selling products from pharmaceutical companies. Practice settings include pharmaceutical companies and telemarketing companies.

EDUCATIONAL REQUIREMENTS
RN preparation is required; some companies prefer a Bachelor of Science in Nursing.

CORE COMPETENCIES/SKILLS NEEDED
- Knowledge of product being promoted
- Ability to manage time effectively
- Good organizational skills
- Marketing skills
- Professional demeanor
- Outgoing personality
- Good communication skills
- Self-motivation
- Ability to be flexible and travel

RELATED WEBSITE AND PROFESSIONAL ORGANIZATION
- Pharmaceutical Representative Online (www.pharmexec.com)

PHARMACEUTICAL RESEARCH NURSE

BASIC DESCRIPTION
The pharmaceutical research nurse is involved in clinical trials that involve the use of pharmacological agents and could be tasked with overseeing the implementation of the research protocol that includes drug handling and dosing in consultation with the pharmacist and clinical researcher.

EDUCATIONAL REQUIREMENTS
RN preparation is required; a Bachelor of Science in Nursing is required in most positions.

CORE COMPETENCIES/SKILLS NEEDED
- Strong phlebotomy skills
- Strong computer and documentation skills
- Excellent interpersonal and communication skills
- Knowledge of research process and Institutional Review Board protocol

RELATED WEBSITE AND PROFESSIONAL ORGANIZATION
- Pharmaceutical Research and Manufacturers of America (www.phrma.org)

PHILANTHROPIST

BASIC DESCRIPTION

Nurse philanthropists are individuals who commit personal and financial resources to create opportunities for a better future. Nurses can get involved by building organizations that support a cause (e.g., an underinsured population that cannot afford health care), supporting a foundation financially and/or with leadership, or volunteering as part of a mission group. The opportunities to become involved in philanthropy are limitless based on an individual's passions or interests.

EDUCATIONAL REQUIREMENTS

There are no educational requirements to become involved in philanthropy. The only requirement is donation of time, skill, or finances.

CORE COMPETENCIES/SKILLS NEEDED

- Ability to commit time, skill, or finance to an organization or foundation supporting a cause
- Passion about nursing, health care, helping others, and promoting wellness for the future
- Selflessness and altruism
- Benevolence and motivation

RELATED WEBSITES AND PROFESSIONAL ORGANIZATIONS

- American Nurses Foundation (www.anfonline.org)
- Philanthropy websites

230

BASIC DESCRIPTION
Plastic and reconstructive surgical nurses care for patients undergoing cosmetic surgery to correct esthetic problems (e.g., face lift, breast augmentation), or to reconstruct some part of the body from disease, accident, or malformations (e.g., skin lesions and tumors, congenital deformities, facial fractures, burns, ulcers, varicose veins, reconstruction after cancer surgery). There is often a great deal of patient happiness and appreciation following the surgery. Opportunities exist to work in hospitals, ambulatory surgery centers, and office practices.

EDUCATIONAL REQUIREMENTS
RN preparation is required. Certification is available as a certified plastic surgical nurse through the Plastic Surgical Nursing Certification Board, Inc.

CORE COMPETENCIES/SKILLS NEEDED
- Skills in patient care
- Specialized skills about the patient's particular operative procedure
- Knowledge of perioperative and postoperative care
- Excellent communication skills
- Consideration of clients' needs

RELATED WEBSITES AND PROFESSIONAL ORGANIZATIONS
- American Society of Plastic Surgical Nurses (www.aspsn.org)
- Plastic Surgical Nursing Certification Board, Inc. (http://psncb.org)

231

POISON INFORMATION NURSE

BASIC DESCRIPTION
Working with poison control centers, the poison information nurse provides education to individuals, organizations, and businesses regarding poison prevention and management.

EDUCATIONAL REQUIREMENTS
RN preparation is required; basic life support certification is required in most positions.

CORE COMPETENCIES/SKILLS NEEDED
- Advanced knowledge of the effects of different types of poison on the body
- Ability to work in a dynamic and high-stress environment, especially for those who are working in emergency departments
- Ability to provide sensitive and empathic care to patients, especially if cause is self-inflicted
- Excellent communication and documentation skills

RELATED WEBSITES AND PROFESSIONAL ORGANIZATIONS
- Agency for Toxic Substances and Disease Registry (www.atsdr.cdc.gov)
- American Academy of Clinical Toxicology (www.clintox.org/index.cfm)
- American Association of Poison Control Centers (www.aapcc.org)

BASIC DESCRIPTION

Politicians are elected officials within a community or political jurisdiction. Nurses have a unique perspective of how health care affects patients and care delivery, and therefore may feel motivated to promote positive changes through policy making. Nurses who aspire to influence health care policy can become involved in politics. In such roles, a nurse can serve the community by acting as an advocate for patients and the nursing profession, proposing policy, influencing implementation of policy, and contributing knowledge in decision making. Nurses can run for office and serve in various elected positions.

EDUCATIONAL REQUIREMENTS

There are constitutional requirements that must be met in order to run for governmental office; however, there is no specific, general educational requirement. An educational background in political science and a health care–related field are preferable.

CORE COMPETENCIES/SKILLS NEEDED

- Honesty and transparency
- Excellent leadership skills
- Confidence and self-assurance
- Decisiveness in making difficult decisions
- Understanding of current state of health care policies
- Critical thinking skills and ability to solve difficult issues
- Motivation, detail orientedness, and focus
- Ability to work independently and as part of a team
- Knowledge of and how to use resources
- Fairness and ability to think and speak objectively

RELATED WEBSITES AND PROFESSIONAL ORGANIZATIONS

- American Association of Colleges of Nursing (www.aacn.nche.edu)
- American Nurses Association (www.nursingworld.org)
- American Nurses Association RN Action (www.rnaction.org)
- State Nurses Associations

233 PRIVATE DUTY NURSE

BASIC DESCRIPTION
Private duty nurses provide total individual patient care in the home or hospital environment with payment coming from a private source or insurance. Private duty nurses can work through an agency or independently.

EDUCATIONAL REQUIREMENTS
RN preparation is required.

CORE COMPETENCIES/SKILLS NEEDED
- Solid foundation in nursing skills
- Ability to assist patients with personal hygiene, activities of daily living, medication management, dressing changes, and intravenous therapy
- Ability to conduct complete assessments and monitoring when necessary
- Ability to provide emotional support
- Problem-solving skills

RELATED WEBSITE AND PROFESSIONAL ORGANIZATION
- New York State Department of Health (www.health.ny.gov/health_care/medicaid/program/longterm/pdn.htm)

PSYCHIATRIC–MENTAL HEALTH NURSE PRACTITIONER

BASIC DESCRIPTION
Psychiatric–mental health nurse practitioners are master's-prepared nurses who focus on behavioral and mental health care of patients. They care for men and women across the life span. They function to diagnose and treat patients with psychiatric illnesses and oversee care in the inpatient and outpatient settings. They also work in mental health facilities or in educational or military institutions.

EDUCATIONAL REQUIREMENTS
RN preparation is required. A Master of Science in Nursing with advanced practice certification as a psychiatric mental health nurse practitioner is required. Certification is available through the American Association of Nurse Practitioners and the American Nurses Credentialing Center. Basic life support and advanced cardiac life support certifications and are also necessary.

CORE COMPETENCIES/SKILLS NEEDED
- Knowledge of mental health and psychiatric illnesses
- Ability to diagnose, treat, and properly refer patients to the appropriate level of treatment with psychiatric disorders
- Excellent interpersonal and communication skills

RELATED WEBSITES AND PROFESSIONAL ORGANIZATIONS
- American Association of Nurse Practitioners (www.aanp.org)
- American Nurses Credentialing Center (www.nursecredentialing.org)
- American Psychiatric Nurses Association (www.apna.org)
- International Society of Psychiatric–Mental Health Nurses (www.ispn-psych.org)

235 PSYCHIATRIC NURSE

BASIC DESCRIPTION

Psychiatric nursing is centered around meeting the health needs of patients, with a particular focus on mental health. Psychiatric nurses may work with patients in an inpatient hospital setting, or a range of outpatient and community-based health care settings. A psychiatric nurse uses therapeutic communication to help patients of all ages better understand themselves and make behavioral changes. Patients who are seen by psychiatric nurses may have a variety of illnesses, such as psychoses, personality and mood disorders, substance abuse disorders, and depression, just to name a few. Psychiatric nurses may work with child, adolescent, or adult patients. Psychiatric nursing involves understanding not only the mental but also the biological aspects of human thought processes and behaviors. Pharmacology also plays a role in psychiatric nursing, because there are many different medications used to treat mental illness and nurses must understand the physiological effects of these medications. Psychiatric nurses may be prepared as advanced practice nurses and as psychotherapists.

EDUCATIONAL REQUIREMENTS

RN preparation is required. Past work experience in any setting where there was a focus on therapeutic communication is extremely important. A solid medical–surgical background with strong assessment experience is important in order to understand and recognize the physiological effects of psychiatric treatment. Certification is available as a psychiatric–mental health nurse, clinical specialist, or nurse practitioner through the American Nurses Credentialing Center; psychiatric nurses may be licensed as individual, family, or group therapists.

CORE COMPETENCIES/SKILLS NEEDED

- Excellent communication skills, because therapeutic communication is used in every encounter with patients
- Strong critical thinking skills
- Ability to work with child, adolescent, adult, and elderly patients
- Observation skills to recognize and understand a patient's nonverbal communication
- Excellent crisis-management skills in order to handle potentially dangerous situations and protect themselves and their patients from harm
- Ability to deal with patients who may be uncooperative or even dangerous at times
- Ability to treat patients with a holistic, nonjudgmental attitude

■ Values for mental health as an important aspect of the health care system
■ Patient advocacy skills

RELATED WEBSITES AND PROFESSIONAL ORGANIZATIONS
■ Alliance for Psychosocial Nursing (www.psychnurse.org)
■ American Academy of Child & Adolescent Psychiatry (http://www.aacap.org)
■ American Nurses Credentialing Center (www.nursingworld.org/ancc/index.htm)
■ American Psychiatric Nurses Association (www.apna.org)

236 PUBLIC AND COMMUNITY HEALTH NURSE

BASIC DESCRIPTION
Public health nurses and community health nurses provide individual and population-focused community-oriented care. Community nurses participate in assessing the population in order to determine needed health services with the goal to improve the overall health of the community through disease prevention, health promotion, and wellness/health education. The public health nurse's goal, in general, is to promote and protect the health of populations using social and public health, public health sciences, and knowledge from nursing. They may also be involved in community health fairs, educational events, and establishing relationships with community organizations. They often assume responsibility for personnel, resources, and patient care in public health and will develop, implement, and evaluate educational programs and activities designed to meet these needs. They may also be involved in one-on-one education, making follow-up phone calls, and conducting home visits, with appropriate documentation of these services. This person may also establish and control the budget and support standards of nursing in the public health practice.

EDUCATIONAL REQUIREMENTS
RN preparation is required. Certification as a community health nurse and as a clinical specialist in community health nursing is available through the American Nurses Credentialing Center.

CORE COMPETENCIES/SKILLS NEEDED
- Knowledge of public health and epidemiology
- Collaborative abilities and team skills
- Assertiveness and self-reliance
- Interpersonal skills
- Analytical skills
- Policy development skills
- Cultural competency
- Management skills
- Must enjoy team effort and providing service in the community

RELATED WEBSITES AND PROFESSIONAL ORGANIZATIONS
- American Nurses Credentialing Center (www.nursecredentialing.org)
- American Public Health Association (www.apha.org)

PUBLIC POLICY ADVISOR

BASIC DESCRIPTION
In this role as a public policy advisor, the nurse provides organizations advice related to health care and policy to achieve goals at the local, regional, or national level.

EDUCATIONAL REQUIREMENTS
RN preparation and at least a master's degree in nursing, health-related field, or health policy.

CORE COMPETENCIES/SKILLS NEEDED
- Knowledge of health policy and legislative process
- Excellent interpersonal and communication skills
- Assertiveness and strong computer skills
- Flexibility with time and ability to travel
- Involvement with various nursing and health care organizations

RELATED WEBSITES AND PROFESSIONAL ORGANIZATIONS
- American Nurses Association (www.ana.org)
- National League for Nursing (www.nln.org)

238 PULMONARY-RESPIRATORY NURSE

BASIC DESCRIPTION
A pulmonary and respiratory nurse promotes pulmonary health for individuals, families, and communities, and cares for persons with pulmonary dysfunction throughout the patient's life span. Respiratory nursing may be preventive, acute, critical, or rehabilitative. There are opportunities to work in hospitals, extended care centers, private companies, health departments, office practices, and clinics.

EDUCATIONAL REQUIREMENTS
RN preparation is required.

CORE COMPETENCIES/SKILLS NEEDED
- Knowledge of respiratory diseases such as asthma, chronic obstructive pulmonary disease, tuberculosis, cystic fibrosis, and respiratory failure
- Excellent patient and family relationships and teaching abilities
- Team skills to work with other members of the health care team
- Ability to deal with issues of grief and loss
- Strong assessment skills
- Knowledge of oxygen therapies, assisted ventilation, and suctioning
- Patience for patient nonadherence to regimen and tobacco abuse
- Ability to discuss smoking cessation techniques, ability to administer and teach pharmacological interventions

RELATED WEBSITES AND PROFESSIONAL ORGANIZATIONS
- American Association of Cardiovascular and Pulmonary Rehabilitation (www.aacvpr.org)
- Respiratory Nursing Society (www.respiratorynursingsociety.org)

QUALITY ASSURANCE NURSE

BASIC DESCRIPTION
Nurses in quality assurance (QA) promote quality and cost-effective outcomes for an organization by interpreting and applying the policies and procedure guidelines. They must identify and coordinate the needs of the patients with needs of the provider and orchestrate patient care among multiple caregivers through the continuum from pre-admission through discharge based on age and cultural and individual patient needs. These nurses support and act as liaisons with the payers, providers, and patients and serve as the primary patient information resource for payers. QA nurses collaborate with physicians and treatment teams to develop patient-care guidelines and serve on quality-improvement teams. There are QA opportunities to work in the private sector, hospitals, and government facilities.

EDUCATIONAL REQUIREMENTS
RN preparation is required. A Bachelor of Science in Nursing is preferred. Certification from the Healthcare Quality Certification Board is available.

CORE COMPETENCIES/SKILLS NEEDED
- Training or experience in utilization review, discharge planning, and case management
- Strong interpersonal and communication skills
- Acute care skills
- Ability to identify problems such as underutilization or overutilization of services
- Self-directed with positive attitude
- Ability to promote and maintain quality care through analysis

RELATED WEBSITES AND PROFESSIONAL ORGANIZATIONS
- Agency for Healthcare Research and Quality (www.ahrq.gov)
- Healthcare Quality Certification Board (www.cphq.org)
- The Joint Commission (www.jointcommission.org)

240   QUALITY DATA ANALYST

BASIC DESCRIPTION

A quality data analyst is responsible for reviewing quality indicators to ensure institutional compliance with quality measures and regulatory standards and reviewing performance with the leaders of the organization. He or she can also be heavily involved in development of measurement mechanisms of data and performance improvement initiatives to ensure patient care standards are met. The quality data analyst is also responsible for collection and tracking of data to ensure that initiatives are effective.

EDUCATIONAL REQUIREMENTS

RN preparation is required. A bachelor's degree in nursing and clinical experience is required. Certification is available.

CORE COMPETENCIES/SKILLS NEEDED

- Ability to communicate effectively
- Ability to interpret, analyze, and synthesize data
- Excellent communication skills
- Ability to work independently
- Consulting skills regarding use of technology
- Ability to utilize various resources to analyze and interpret variances and make comparisons with national and regional benchmarks
- Ability to manage multiple priorities
- Knowledge of quality improvement processes and data measurement

RELATED WEBSITES AND PROFESSIONAL ORGANIZATIONS

- American Medical Informatics Association (www.amia.org)
- American Nursing Credentialing Center (www.nursecredentialing.org)
- American Nursing Informatics Association (www.ania.org)

QUALITY DIRECTOR

BASIC DESCRIPTION
A quality director is a nurse leader who is responsible for oversight of hospital or health system quality performance. Responsibilities include leading the organization in a multidisciplinary core measure process, setting strategic goals, monitoring data of quality metrics, and developing performance improvement plans accordingly. Furthermore, quality directors lead the hospital in preparation for and execution of regulatory agency surveys by ensuring that standards are met. Additionally, they are available to provide consultation services to departments to assist them in achieving quality metric goals.

EDUCATIONAL REQUIREMENTS
A bachelor's degree in nursing or another health care–related field is required. A master's degree in a health care–related field or nursing is preferred. Certification options, such as certified professional in health care quality (CPHQ) or certified professional in infection control, are available and highly preferred.

CORE COMPETENCIES/SKILLS NEEDED
- Ability to collect, analyze, synthesize, interpret, and present data
- Excellent leadership skills
- Thorough knowledge of regulatory agency standards and accreditation process
- Understanding of finances and budgeting
- Ability to manage multiple projects at the same time
- Ability to educate and assess understanding of staff
- Skill in computer programs
- Ability to work independently and as part of a team
- Understanding of clinical and hospital operations
- Effective communication and interpersonal skills
- Attention to detail
- Ability to develop and initiate performance improvement plans to improve hospital performance
- Ability to promote and maintain quality care through analysis
- Ability to identify problems and identify processes for improvement

RELATED WEBSITES AND PROFESSIONAL ORGANIZATIONS
- Center for Improvement in Healthcare Quality (www.cihq.org)
- National Association for Healthcare Quality (www.nahq.org)
- National Committee for Quality Assurance (www.ncqa.org)
- The Joint Commission (www.jointcommission.org)

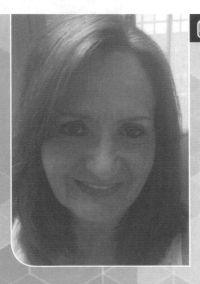

1. What is your educational background in nursing (and other areas) and what formal credentials do you hold?

I was educated in a hybrid program between a diploma and a baccalaureate degree program. My clinical nursing and science courses were in the diploma program and I took exams for college credit. My liberal arts, languages, and nursing leadership courses were at college. I was able to complete my Bachelor of Science in Nursing on a part-time basis. I continued my academic education, receiving a Master of Art in Nursing with an education and leadership focus. I am currently enrolled in a Doctor of Nursing Practice program. I have American Nurses Credentialing Center (ANCC) certification in pediatric nursing. I completed the professional development program of the Institute for Healthcare Improvement Advisor.

2. How did you first become interested in your current career?

My interest in quality, patient outcomes, and professional practice started early in my professional career. I participated in peer review and concurrent auditing of care as a staff nurse. As I advanced in my career, I led peer review teams, nursing and interdisciplinary. In leadership positions, I directed care and practice in very regulated clinical areas: dialysis, behavioral health, and opioid treatment. My main clinical specialization is women's and children's health care. The obstetrics service was in an urban area whose population was high risk, with many comorbidities and poor health habits. Obstetrics is an area of practice with high legal liability. Thus, it was first to focus on creating a culture of safety, implementing TeamSTEPPS, simulation and safe

Continued

practices learned from aviation. I colead an obstetrics safety team, collaboratively creating a culture of safety for patients to be cared for and for providers to administer care. The realized improvement in outcomes spurred us to continue this journey. At this time, the health care environment was changing and outcomes were being shared with the public. Health care organizations were being measured on outcomes of care and ratings were published by several groups (Leapfrog [www.leapfrog.com], Centers for Medicare & Medicaid Services, hospital compare.gov, American Heart Association, *Consumer Reports*, *U.S. News & World Report*, and others). In nursing, we also became transparent with outcomes and benchmarking with local and national standards. The Magnet™ program was initiated. Outcomes of care are essential to achieve and sustain Magnet certification. The National Database for Nursing Quality Indicators was initiated and has become the standard.

3. What are the most rewarding aspects of your career?

In my role I have developed, through education and coaching, unit-based quality champions among frontline staff, professional nurses, and unlicensed assistive personnel. To witness their development and keen interest in improving patient outcomes and reducing patient harm is a rewarding aspect of my career. Professional peer review is rewarding as staff own practice in that process. I have observed staff improving their own practice and documentation by participating in peer review, concurrent audits, and evaluating evidence-based practice. The achiever in me feels rewarded when targets are bested and goals achieved. Ultimately it is the patient who benefits and that is core to why I became a nurse.

4. What advice would you give to someone contemplating the same path in nursing?

My advice is to get involved, participate in care audits, performance improvement teams, and research. Expand your knowledge by attending conferences, reading quality journals (*Journal of Nursing Care Quality*, *Journal of Healthcare Quality*), joining professional nursing associations, and enrolling in educational programs focusing on health care quality. Through these activities, it is very important to network with colleagues and share your professional interests and expertise. The American Nurses Association has an annual Quality, Safety, and Staffing conference. The Institute for Healthcare Improvement has an annual conference. Professional associations with a specific focus on health care quality are American Society for Quality (ASQ) and the National Association for Healthcare Quality (NAHQ). Lastly, consider obtaining certification as a certified professional in health care quality.

242 QUALITY IMPROVEMENT SPECIALIST/MANAGER

BASIC DESCRIPTION

A quality improvement specialist or quality improvement manager works under a quality director to carry out quality assurance programs and performance improvement plans in a health care organization. The quality improvement specialists work collaboratively with a multidisciplinary team to collect data and coordinate and implement performance improvement plans. They also work with frontline clinical staff to educate them on strategies and initiatives to improve performance, and track compliance to meet quality goals. Additionally, they assist with preparation of surveys for accreditation or regulatory agencies.

EDUCATIONAL REQUIREMENTS

A bachelor's degree in nursing or a health care–related field is required. A master's degree in nursing or a health care–related field is highly preferred. Certification options as certified professional in health care quality or Certified Profession in Infection Control are available and highly preferred.

CORE COMPETENCIES/SKILLS NEEDED

- Ability to collect, analyze, synthesize, interpret, and present data
- Excellent leadership skills
- Thorough knowledge in regulatory agency standards and accreditation process
- Understanding of finances and budgeting
- Ability to manage multiple projects at the same time
- Ability to educate and assess understanding of staff
- Skill in computer programs
- Ability to work independently and as part of a team
- Understanding of clinical and hospital operations
- Effective communication and interpersonal skills
- Detail oriented
- Ability to develop and initiate performance improvement plans to improve hospital performance
- Ability to promote and maintain quality care through analysis
- Ability to identify problems and identify processes for improvement

RELATED WEBSITES AND PROFESSIONAL ORGANIZATIONS

- Center for Improvement in Healthcare Quality (www.cihq.org)
- National Association for Healthcare Quality (www.nahq.org)
- National Committee for Quality Assurance (www.ncqa.org)
- The Joint Commission (www.jointcommission.org)

243 RADIATION–ONCOLOGY NURSE

BASIC DESCRIPTION
The nurse practicing radiation oncology is a pivotal care team member who assists patients throughout the course of treatment and beyond completion of therapy. As this is a growing field, these nurses need to be prepared to assess, intervene, educate, and advocate for their patients during treatment. They also provide emotional support and help patients navigate the medical system after treatment to ensure follow-up care for continued survival.

EDUCATIONAL REQUIREMENTS
RN preparation is required; a bachelor's degree in nursing with certification in the field of oncology is preferred.

CORE COMPETENCIES/SKILLS NEEDED
- Current knowledge of various types of cancer and their treatments
- Knowledge of chemotherapy and surgical interventions for cancer
- Competency in radiation biology, physics, safety, and side effects
- Critical thinking skills
- Sensitivity to patient needs and concerns
- Ability to teach patients and families

RELATED WEBSITES AND PROFESSIONAL ORGANIZATIONS
- American Society for Radiation Oncology (www.astro.org)
- Association for Pediatric Oncology Nurses (www.apon.org)
- Oncology Nursing Society (www.ons.org)

RADIATION–ONCOLOGY NURSE PRACTITIONER

BASIC DESCRIPTION
Radiation–oncology nurse practitioners work directly with a radiation oncologist to provide radiation treatment to patients with cancer. Their role is to assess patients, order and interpret diagnostic tests, assist with development of a treatment plan, manage symptoms and side effects, prescribe medications, assist with performing certain procedures, educate patients, and ensure adequate follow-up care.

EDUCATIONAL REQUIREMENTS
RN preparation is required. A Master of Science in Nursing with advanced practice certification as a nurse practitioner is required. Certification is available through the American Association of Nurse Practitioners and the American Nurses Credentialing Center. Basic life support and advanced cardiac life support certifications are also necessary. It is recommended to have specialized training in oncology as well.

CORE COMPETENCIES/SKILLS NEEDED
- Extensive knowledge of various types of cancer and their treatments
- Expertise in radiation biology, physics, safety, and side effects
- Ability to interpret diagnostic testing and develop treatment plan
- Ability to assist in performing treatments and procedures
- Sensitivity to patient needs and concerns
- Strong teaching skills for patients and families

RELATED WEBSITES AND PROFESSIONAL ORGANIZATIONS
- American Association of Nurse Practitioners (www.aanp.org)
- American Nurses Credentialing Center (www.nursecredentialing.org)
- American Society for Radiation Oncology (www.astro.org)
- Association for Pediatric Oncology Nurses (www.apon.org)
- Oncology Nursing Society (www.ons.org)

245 RADIOLOGY NURSE

BASIC DESCRIPTION
Radiology nurses work primarily in the hospital setting, assisting, performing, and teaching in the area of radiological imaging. Contemporary radiology departments are equipped with state-of-the-art imaging capacities, and radiology nurses assist in the care of patients undergoing invasive procedures.

EDUCATIONAL REQUIREMENTS
RN preparation is required. Certification is available from the Radiologic Nursing Certification Board, Inc.

CORE COMPETENCIES/SKILLS NEEDED
- Strong anatomy and physiology theory base and education in disease processes of human body
- Technical proficiency and knowledge of procedures to be performed
- Good teaching skills to prepare and help clients reach best outcome from a test/procedure
- Good knowledge of body mechanics for optimal positioning of patient for procedure
- Ability to identify and interpret life-threatening arrhythmias
- Skill in reviewing patient's clinical history for potential indicators that might contraindicate the procedure
- Skills in advocating for patient safety

RELATED WEBSITES AND PROFESSIONAL ORGANIZATIONS
- Radiologic Nursing Certification Board, Inc. (www.arinursing.org/certification)
- Radiological Society of North American (www.rsna.org)

RAPID RESPONSE NURSE

BASIC DESCRIPTION

Rapid response nurses are part of an expert clinical team in the acute care area, whose main goal is to prevent deaths and arrest hemodynamic decline in patients outside of intensive care units. They are experts in assessment and have clinical skills in implementing early interventions to prevent cardiopulmonary arrest.

EDUCATIONAL REQUIREMENTS

RN preparation, basic life support, and advanced cardiac life support certifications are required.

CORE COMPETENCIES/SKILLS NEEDED

- Excellent assessment and critical thinking skills
- Excellent clinical skills, such as initiating intravenous access, defibrillation, and suctioning
- Ability to work in a highly dynamic environment and to quickly respond to urgent calls anywhere in the acute care facility
- Excellent communication skills while working with other members of the rapid response team

RELATED WEBSITES AND PROFESSIONAL ORGANIZATIONS

- Institute for Healthcare Improvement (www.ihi.org/resources/Pages/ ImprovementStories/RapidResponseTeamsReducingCodesandRaisingMorale .aspx)
- Rapid Response Systems (psnet.ahrq.gov/primers/primer/4/ rapid-response-systems)

247 RECOVERY ROOM NURSE

BASIC DESCRIPTION
As a highly skilled clinician, the recovery room nurse is responsible for monitoring immediate postoperative patients across age groups. He or she works in varied health care settings such as acute care facilities and ambulatory care settings. The recovery room nurse is also responsible for ensuring that acute complications arising from surgery are prevented by intervening if acute life-threatening complications occur.

EDUCATIONAL REQUIREMENTS
RN preparation is required. Basic life support and advanced cardiac life support certifications are required; certification is available from the American Board of Perianesthesia Nursing Certification.

CORE COMPETENCIES/SKILLS NEEDED
- Excellent communication and assessment skills
- Knowledge of cardiovascular and respiratory physiology and pathophysiology, and critical care concepts
- Ability to make quick decisions regarding patient's clinical condition and make urgent referrals to physicians
- Ability to work under pressure
- Knowledge of telemetry and ventilator management

RELATED WEBSITES AND PROFESSIONAL ORGANIZATIONS
- American Board of Perianesthesia Nursing Certification, Inc. (www.cpancapa.org)
- American Society of PeriAnesthesia Nurses (www.aspan.org)
- Preoperative Association (www.pre-op.org)

BASIC DESCRIPTION
Nurse recruiters develop and implement short- and long-term recruitment plans and strategies to meet nurse staffing needs. They also create, coordinate, and maintain a wide range of cost-effective recruitment strategies to generate applicant pools and hires. Work settings include hospitals, nursing homes, schools of nursing, and travel health care companies.

EDUCATIONAL REQUIREMENTS
RN preparation is required.

CORE COMPETENCIES/SKILLS NEEDED
- Excellent interpersonal skills
- Ability to screen and interview prospective job applicants
- Ability to develop relationships with the various nursing programs/schools in the area to promote nursing career opportunities and market
- Ability to contact, interview, and place nurses in jobs at a health care facility
- Self-direction and self-motivation
- Team skills
- Marketing skills
- Excellent phone voice, positive and enthusiastic
- Organizational skills
- Focus with attention to detail

RELATED WEBSITES AND PROFESSIONAL ORGANIZATIONS
- National Association for Health Care Recruitment (www.nahcr.com)
- Nurse Recruiter for Nurses by Nurses (www.nurserecruiter.com)

249 REHABILITATION NURSE

BASIC DESCRIPTION

Rehabilitation nursing is a specialty practice area that involves care of individuals with altered functional ability and altered lifestyle. Rehabilitation nurses begin to work with injured or ill individuals and their families soon after a disabling injury or chronic illness strikes, and they continue to provide support after these individuals go home or return to work or school. The goal of rehabilitation nursing is to assist individuals with disabilities and chronic illness in the restoration, maintenance, and promotion of optimal health. Rehabilitation nursing practice occurs in many settings and involves a variety of roles. Most opportunities exist in hospitals (including specialty hospitals), long-term care facilities, and free-standing facilities.

EDUCATIONAL REQUIREMENTS

RN preparation is required. An RN with at least 2 years of practice in rehabilitation nursing can earn distinction as a certified rehabilitation registered nurse (CRRN) by successfully completing an examination that validates expertise. Likewise, an RN with a CRRN and a master's degree or doctorate in nursing can earn certification as a CRRN-advanced.

CORE COMPETENCIES/SKILLS NEEDED

- Long-term patient-and-colleague relationships
- Ability to work with clients from infancy to elderly
- Teamwork and collaboration capability
- Patient and family education
- Innovative thinking
- Autonomy and independence
- Skill at treating alterations in functional ability and lifestyle resulting from injury, disability, and chronic illness
- Skill in providing comfort, therapy, and education
- Skill to promote health-conducive adjustments, support adaptive capabilities, and promote achievable independence
- Skill in promoting holistic, comprehensive, and compassionate end-of-life care, including promotion of comfort and relief from pain
- Excellent functional assessment skills
- Skill in team management acting as multisystem integrators and team leaders, working with physicians, therapists, and others to solve problems and promote patients' maximal independence

- Ability to work with others to adapt ongoing care to the resources available, which distinguishes the practice of rehabilitation nursing
- Goal orientedness and focus on helping patients return to optimal functionality
- Ability to provide holistic care to meet patients' medical, vocational, educational, environmental, and spiritual needs
- Ability to function not only as caregivers but also as coordinators, collaborators, counselors, and case managers

RELATED WEBSITE AND PROFESSIONAL ORGANIZATION
- Association of Rehabilitation Nurses (www.rehabnurse.org)

250 REPRODUCTIVE MEDICINE NURSE PRACTITIONER

BASIC DESCRIPTION
A reproductive medicine nurse practitioner is an advanced practice nurse who focuses on fertility and treatments for infertility. He or she works with a team of medical professionals to provide treatment for women experiencing fertility issues. The nurse practitioner (NP) is responsible for history taking and physical exam, consultation, performing imaging and diagnostic testing, collaborating with a physician to discuss treatment options, performing treatments, and providing ongoing monitoring and counseling. He or she may also perform procedures such as in vitro fertilization (IVF) and intrauterine insemination (IUI). Employment is typically found in fertility clinics, women's health clinics, or private practice.

EDUCATIONAL REQUIREMENTS
RN preparation is required. A Master of Science in Nursing with advanced practice certification as an NP is required. Certification is available through the American Association of Nurse Practitioners and the American Nurses Credentialing Center. Basic life support and advanced cardiac life support certifications are also necessary. A certificate course is available through the American Society for Reproductive Medicine.

CORE COMPETENCIES/SKILLS NEEDED
- Sensitivity to patient needs and concerns
- Knowledge about women's health, infertility, and treatments
- Ability to be patient with clients throughout fertility process
- Excellent history-taking and physical exam skills
- Excellent interpersonal skills and ability to connect with patients
- Excellent communication and counseling skills
- Ability to collaborate and work as part of a team

RELATED WEBSITES AND PROFESSIONAL ORGANIZATIONS
- American Association of Nurse Practitioners (www.aanp.org)
- American Nurses Credentialing Center (www.nursecredentialing.org)
- American Society for Reproductive Medicine (www.asrm.org)

REPRODUCTIVE NURSE

BASIC DESCRIPTION
A reproductive nurse provides education and counseling to individuals and their families about fertility concerns and other reproduction-related concerns that include menopause, impotence, and other forms of sexual dysfunctions.

EDUCATIONAL REQUIREMENTS
RN preparation is required.

CORE COMPETENCIES/SKILLS NEEDED
- Sensitivity to patients and their families
- Excellent verbal and written communication skills
- Advanced knowledge of the reproductive system physiology, pathophysiology, and disease management
- Strong computer skills and knowledge of electronic health record documentation

RELATED WEBSITES AND PROFESSIONAL ORGANIZATIONS
- American Society for Reproductive Medicine (www.asrm.org)
- Association of Reproductive Health Professionals (www.arhp.org)
- North American Menopause Society (www.menopause.org)

252 RESEARCH AND INNOVATION DIRECTOR

BASIC DESCRIPTION

A research and innovation director supervises nursing practice and education in a health care organization. He or she is ultimately responsible for the nursing department in regards to performing, analyzing, and sharing evidence-based research into practice to improve practice and ensure quality patient outcomes. He or she works to develop and innovate clinical practice guidelines and care interventions that incorporate this knowledge in decision making and patient care.

EDUCATION REQUIREMENTS

RN preparation is required. A bachelor's degree in nursing is necessary. A master's degree in nursing or a health care–related field is preferable. A doctorate-level degree is highly desired. Experience in a leadership or managerial role is required.

CORE COMPETENCIES/SKILLS NEEDED

- Excellent leadership and management skills
- Passion for research
- Ability to communicate effectively
- Skill in collecting, analyzing, interpreting, and disseminating data and information
- Analytical and organizational skills
- Knowledge of and skills in research methods
- Writing and reporting skills, including proposal development skills
- Ability to work under pressure
- Skill in managing teams
- Ability to work collaboratively as part of a team and independently

RELATED WEBSITES AND ORGANIZATIONS

- National Institute of Nursing Research; a branch of the U.S. Health and Human Services National Institutes of Health (www.ninr.nih.gov)
- National Institutes of Health, Understanding Clinical Trials (https://clinicaltrials.gov/ct2/info/understand)

BASIC DESCRIPTION

A research coordinator performs a role that includes coordination and management, and conducts clinical research under the supervision of a designated investigator. The research coordinator position may be undertaken with a wide range of scientific investigations (e.g., basic research, clinical research, and epidemiological research) under the direction of scientists from many health disciplines.

EDUCATIONAL REQUIREMENTS

RN preparation is required. Undergraduate and graduate preparation and a background in participation in research are desirable.

CORE COMPETENCIES/SKILLS NEEDED

- Knowledge of the research process
- Knowledge of the ethical requirements for conducting research and knowledge of the human subjects research requirements
- Organizational skills
- Writing and reporting skills, including proposal development skills to assist the investigator in preparing proposals and reports
- Ability to work under pressure to accomplish research goals
- Knowledge of potential funding agency requirements
- Skill at managing teams including data collectors, research assistants, and project investigators

RELATED WEBSITE AND PROFESSIONAL ORGANIZATION

- National Institutes of Health, Understanding Clinical Trials (https://clinicaltrials.gov/ct2/info/understand)

254 RESEARCHER

BASIC DESCRIPTION

A nurse researcher conducts studies related to individual, family, and community health; symptoms of illness; nursing interventions to promote health and decrease incidence or symptoms of illness; and conducts research related to nursing and health care delivery including workforce planning. The research may involve a large project funded through the National Institutes of Health or a small project supported by funds from the researcher's institution. Research requires an attention to detail; thus, the work is methodical and sometimes tedious. Researchers may work alone or in teams with other nurse researchers or clinicians; often the research undertaken by nurse scientists is multidisciplinary in nature, thus requiring the researchers to engage in team building and team functioning. Researchers often work under great pressure to meet deadlines for funding agencies or publication deadlines.

EDUCATIONAL REQUIREMENTS

A PhD degree in nursing or related discipline is required.

CORE COMPETENCIES/SKILLS NEEDED

- Knowledge of and skills in research methods
- Knowledge of statistical methods and analyses
- Grant-writing skills
- Analytical and organizational skills
- Writing skills
- Team-building skills

RELATED WEBSITES AND PROFESSIONAL ORGANIZATIONS

- National Institute of Nursing Research; a branch of the U.S. Health and Human Services National Institutes of Health (www.ninr.nih.gov)
- Sigma Theta Tau International (www.nursingsociety.org)

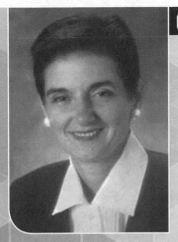

PROFILE: MARY KERR

Nurse Researcher

1. What is your educational background in nursing (and other areas) and what formal credentials do you hold?

I have a diploma in nursing, a Bachelor of Science (BSN) and a Master of Science in Nursing, and a PhD.

2. How did you first become interested in the career that you are currently in?

I became interested in nursing in high school, and was a member of the Future Nurses of America club. I became interested in research when I conducted a research project as part of my BSN—I counted microbes on gloves used in the operating room. I was intrigued by the idea of using data to examine and improve the outcomes of clinical care.

3. What are the most rewarding aspects of your career?

Each position that I held offered different rewards. Conducting research within an interdisciplinary, clinical environment was extremely challenging and intellectually stimulating. I also enjoyed teaching in an academic environment, helping students learn how to solve clinical problems by using data. Moving from academia to government was a fascinating change—now, as deputy director of the National Institute of Nursing Research (NINR), I get to see the benefits of nursing science applied to the health of the public on a national scale, which is deeply rewarding and enlightening. Throughout my career as a scientist, I have devoted myself to the training and mentoring of the next generation of investigators. It has been

Continued

PROFILE: MARY KERR
Continued

most gratifying to work for a public institution that shares this goal and devotes a significant percentage of its resources toward developing new investigators.

4. What advice would you give to someone contemplating the same career path in nursing?

First, I would strongly recommend that, as freshmen, undergraduate nursing students participate in a research project headed by a nurse scientist. Whether they volunteer or are hired as student workers, the experience will help them determine if they might want to pursue a career as a nurse scientist. If they are interested in that path, the second step is to apply to a PhD program in nursing research before they graduate. Next, rather than working full time and going to school part time, like the majority of nurses who seek advanced degrees, I would advise them to attend school full time and work as a nurse part time. This way everything they learn while pursuing their advanced degree will be integrated into their clinical practice.

To those who are already practicing nurses, I would encourage them to consider research, even if it means returning to school. Nursing science is coming into its own and, given the looming nurse faculty shortages, the field is wide open. Nurses, with their training in clinical observation and evaluation of patients, already have the basic skills that are critical for a research career; it is a natural next step to improve outcomes and help patients via research. Despite what many believe, pursuing a research career does not necessarily mean leaving patients behind. On the contrary, developing research projects with real-world benefits often requires regular interaction with patients. I encourage anyone who is interested in learning more about this field to visit the NINR website, which offers a condensed introductory nursing research course.

RESPIRATORY NURSE PRACTITIONER 255

BASIC DESCRIPTION
Respiratory nurse practitioners deal with patients across age groups who have acute or chronic pulmonary disorders, such as asthma, chronic obstructive pulmonary disorders, and cystic fibrosis. They work in various health care practice settings. Aside from providing primary care, they also educate patients with regard to prevention of future attacks and complications and participate in health promotion and maintenance activities.

EDUCATIONAL REQUIREMENTS
RN preparation and nurse practitioner certification are required. Basic life support and advanced cardiac life support certifications are required for most positions.

CORE COMPETENCIES/SKILLS NEEDED
- Knowledge of anatomy, physiology, and pathophysiology of the respiratory system and their common treatments
- Excellent assessment and communication skills
- Knowledge of educational principles, and experience in public speaking are highly desirable

RELATED WEBSITES AND PROFESSIONAL ORGANIZATIONS
- American Association of Cardiovascular and Pulmonary Rehabilitation (www.aacvpr.org)
- Association of Respiratory Nurse Specialists (arns.co.uk)

256 RHEUMATOLOGY NURSE

BASIC DESCRIPTION
Rheumatology nurses provide care for patients suffering from diseases, such as arthritis, fibromyalgia, and myositis, that affect muscles, bones, and joints. Their goals are to provide interventions to relieve pain and prevent complications, and to educate patients about health-promoting behaviors to decrease pain symptoms and prevent complications. They work in various health care settings, such as acute care facilities, ambulatory centers, and specialized rheumatology clinics.

EDUCATIONAL REQUIREMENTS
RN preparation and basic life support certification are required.

CORE COMPETENCIES/SKILLS NEEDED
- Knowledge of evidence-based approaches to pain management
- Excellent assessment and communication skills
- Strong leadership and organizational skills, as rheumatology nurses could assume managerial responsibilities when working in ambulatory centers
- Excellent technical nursing skills such as phlebotomy skills

RELATED WEBSITES AND PROFESSIONAL ORGANIZATIONS
- American College of Rheumatology (www.rheumatology.org)
- Arthritis Foundation (www.arthritis.org)
- Rheumatology Nurses Society (www.rns-network.org)

RISK CONTROL COORDINATOR

BASIC DESCRIPTION
Risk control coordinators are responsible for the assessment, planning, implementation, and evaluation of risk control activities, and coordinator of a hospital or health care facility's performance improvement program. They are accountable for day-to-day risk management issues. This person typically works under the risk control manager or director in an organization.

EDUCATIONAL REQUIREMENTS
A bachelor's degree in a health care–related field is required. In some cases, a master's degree in a health-related field is required. RN preparation is not required, but is an excellent educational background for risk management.

CORE COMPETENCIES/SKILLS NEEDED
- Knowledge of government regulations
- Thorough understanding of organization's policies and procedures
- Strong writing skills
- Excellent verbal and written communication skills
- Strong assessment skills
- Ability to be organized and attentive to detail
- Ability to analyze complex situations
- Ability to handle stress and difficult decisions

RELATED WEBSITES AND PROFESSIONAL ORGANIZATIONS
- Agency for Healthcare Research and Quality (www.ahrq.gov)
- American Society for Healthcare Risk Management (www.ashrm.org)
- Risk Management Society (www.rims.org)
- The Joint Commission (www.jointcommission.org)

258

RISK MANAGEMENT NURSE

BASIC DESCRIPTION
Risk management nurses have special knowledge and interest in the work environment of nurses and the injuries nurses sustain as a result of environmental exposures. They may be consultants responsible for reviewing medical records, policies, and procedures, and thus would be aware of legal aspects and their implications. Risk management nurses conduct programs covering the aspects of documentation and internal procedures in order to protect patients and staff from injuries.

EDUCATIONAL REQUIREMENTS
RN preparation is required.

CORE COMPETENCIES/SKILLS NEEDED
- Ability to provide objective view of environment in relation to patient and nurse safety
- Computer skills
- Analytical skills
- Communication skills
- Ability to handle multiple tasks simultaneously
- Sharp visual acuity
- Keen judgment
- Excellent observational skills
- Strong assessment skills

RELATED WEBSITES AND PROFESSIONAL ORGANIZATIONS
- Agency for Healthcare Research and Quality (www.ahrq.gov)
- American Nurses Association (www.ana.org)
- The Joint Commission (www.jointcommission.org)

RURAL HEALTH NURSE 259

BASIC DESCRIPTION

A rural health nurse is a generalist who practices professional nursing in communities with relatively low populations that are geographically and often culturally isolated. Rural nurses have close ties to and interaction with the communities in which they practice and often practice with a great deal of autonomy and independence. A strong and varied experience base is crucial in rural nursing, as the population that the rural nurse must care for will range from infants to the elderly. Therefore, a rural nurse must know about every stage of life. Experience with rural communities is a benefit in order to understand the cultural context within which the people live. For most rural nurses, traveling between isolated communities is part of their role. Rural nurses may operate from a clinic or small hospital, while others may base themselves out of a large mobile health center.

EDUCATIONAL REQUIREMENTS

RN preparation is required.

CORE COMPETENCIES/SKILLS NEEDED

- Physical assessment and emergency/trauma management skills
- Skill in all areas of nursing, with clinical and assessment skills that reflect this proficiency
- Critical care skills
- Aptitude for teaching
- Wide knowledge of resources within the community
- Management skills
- Surgical, obstetric, and intravenous therapy skills; ability to operate and troubleshoot equipment is useful
- Knowledge about the areas, such as pharmaceuticals, and the region in which one is practicing, as well as an in-depth awareness of cultural norms and values
- Ability to adapt to the resources that are available
- Ability to use innovative and creative solutions to the challenges that exist in locations without major medical centers
- Ability to practice independently, even without the supplies and equipment available that one needs
- Ability to value the close interaction they have with the individuals, families, and communities they serve

RELATED WEBSITE AND PROFESSIONAL ORGANIZATION

- Rural Nursing Organization (www.rno.org)

260 SCHOOL NURSE

BASIC DESCRIPTION
The school nurse practices professional nursing within an educational setting with the goal of assisting students to develop to their greatest physical, emotional, and intellectual ability. School nurses promote health and safety practices and provide interventions to actual and potential health problems. These nurses respond to acute injuries within the school population, as well as assist students to manage chronic conditions, such as food allergies, asthma, and other illnesses. Practice settings include school systems, state health departments, and county health departments.

EDUCATIONAL REQUIREMENTS
RN preparation is required. Some school systems and/or health departments now require that school nurses have baccalaureate or master's degrees in nursing. Certification is available from the National Board for Certification of School Nurses.

CORE COMPETENCIES/SKILLS NEEDED
- General experience with children
- Strong foundation in physical assessment and first aid and emergency care
- Solid skill base and understanding of pediatric medicine
- Knowledge of developmental stages in order to provide age-appropriate care
- Strong communication and interpersonal skills to assess and determine the health care needs of the children and their families
- Computer skills to chart and track students' records and immunization status
- Ability to relate to children and communicate with patients and the school community
- Ability to provide health education
- Medication management of children while they are in school
- Skill to participate as a member of a multidisciplinary educational team and collaborate with other members of the educational environment
- Ability to provide care for minor ailments such as a scraped knee as well as potentially serious conditions such as an allergic reaction or a major injury
- Ensure the safety and well-being of all the children in the school
- Ability to deal with issues such as school violence, suicide, and unwanted teen pregnancies

RELATED WEBSITES AND PROFESSIONAL ORGANIZATIONS

- National Association of School Nurses (www.nasn.org)
- National Association of State School Nurse Consultants (www.nassnc.org)
- National Board for Certification of School Nurses (www.nbcsn.org)

26 | SCIENTIST

BASIC DESCRIPTION

These nurses lead scientific research opportunities in nursing and health care in their employing institutions in a variety of potential areas of specialty. In turn, their work improves nursing care by advancing evidence-based practice. Applying for grants to fund projects is an important aspect of a scientist's role.

EDUCATIONAL REQUIREMENTS

RN preparation and bachelor's degree in nursing are required.

CORE COMPETENCIES/SKILLS NEEDED

- Knowledge of scientific method and grant application process
- Ability to synthesize, analyze, and interpret data
- Excellent writing skills
- Creative and innovative thought process
- Focus and ability to meet deadlines
- Strong organizational skills
- Excellent communication skills

RELATED WEBSITE AND PROFESSIONAL ORGANIZATION

- National Institute of Nursing Research (www.ninr.nih.gov)

PROFILE: **RONALD HICKMAN**

Nurse Scientist

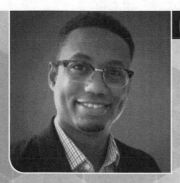

1. What is your educational background in nursing (and other areas) and what formal credentials do you hold?

I hold four degrees: Bachelor of Arts (BA) in Biological Science, Master of Nursing (MN), Master of Science in Nursing (MSN), and PhD in Nursing Science. After completion of my doctoral education, I completed 4 years of postdoctoral training in multidisciplinary clinical and translational science. I hold a certification from the American Nurses Credentialing Center as an acute care nurse practitioner and have more than 15 years of nursing experience.

2. How did you first become interested in your current career?

My interest in becoming a nurse scientist is grounded in my experiences as a critical care nurse. Early in my professional nursing career, I found myself asking questions that often centered on how to improve the quality of care for critically ill patients and their families. I sought mentors in experienced nurse and physician colleagues who encouraged my curiosity and inspired me to further pursue graduate nursing education. Given my interest in inquiry derived from my clinical practice, I enrolled in an MSN program focusing on the management of acutely and critically ill patients and their family systems. My graduate nursing experience expanded my perspective on the clinical management of acutely and critically ill patients but also exposed me to doctorally prepared nurse scientists and advanced practice nurses who were systematically solving clinically relevant problems. As a result, I was inspired to pursue a PhD in nursing science and develop a research program that holds the promise to improve the outcomes of the critically ill and their families. My career as a nurse scientist has helped to establish an evidence base that is used by stakeholders to shape institutional and national policies for patients and families contemplating health and health care choices.

Continued

3. What are the most rewarding aspects of your career?

As a nurse scientist, there are several rewarding aspects of this career. I find the advancement of nursing and health science a reward that affords endless opportunities. Through the conduct and dissemination of research, I have been able to shape nursing practice, science, and health policy. The rewards of choosing a career as a nurse scientist extend beyond the immediate gratifications of the nurse–patient interaction toward far-reaching change that can significantly influence the health of Americans nationwide.

4. What advice would you give to someone contemplating the same career path in nursing?

The key to a successful career as a nurse scientist is self-awareness and perseverance. A career as a nurse scientist often entails delayed reward. Periodic reflection is needed to become self-aware of the tensions that can manifest between the immediate gratifications of a clinical nursing career and the delayed rewards of choosing a career as a nurse scientist. I would advise someone contemplating a career as a nurse scientist to be introspective and practice perseverance along this journey.

SCRUB NURSE

BASIC DESCRIPTION

The scrub nurse is part of the perioperative surgical team. He or she works side by side with the surgeon during the intraoperative phase. The scrub nurse observes strict aseptic technique while providing and anticipating the need for sterile surgical equipment such as scalpels, forceps, and sponges that the surgeon needs during the procedure.

EDUCATIONAL REQUIREMENTS

RN preparation is highly preferred; basic life support certification is required.

CORE COMPETENCIES/SKILLS NEEDED

- Excellent communication skills
- Ability to anticipate the needs of the surgeon
- Knowledge of surgical asepsis

RELATED WEBSITE AND PROFESSIONAL ORGANIZATION

- Association of Operating Room Nurses (www.aorn.org)

263

SERVICE LINE ADMINISTRATOR/ NURSING DIRECTOR

BASIC DESCRIPTION

A nursing service line administrator (or nursing director) is a nurse leader who reports to the chief nursing officer or vice president of nursing in a hospital or health care system. He or she is accountable for directing nursing operations within a service line, such as medicine, surgery, perioperative, or cardiovascular. This involves leading the development, implementation, and assessment of quality patient care in line with the institution's mission, vision and values as well as regulatory standards. In this role, nursing service line administrators also collaborate with interdisciplinary teams to ensure safe, efficient patient care. They directly oversee the work of unit-based nursing leaders.

EDUCATIONAL REQUIREMENTS

RN preparation is required. A bachelor's degree in nursing is necessary, but a master's degree in nursing or a doctorate degree is preferred. Certification is available through the American Organization of Nurse Executives.

CORE COMPETENCIES/SKILLS NEEDED

- Excellent leadership skills
- Strong communication and interpersonal skills
- Attentiveness and decisiveness
- Creativity with critical thinking skills
- Ability to collaborate and work as a team or as an individual
- Ability to analyze and synthesize data and information
- Thorough knowledge of hospital policies and regulatory agency standards
- Understanding of finances and budgeting
- Ability to promote professional nursing practice

RELATED WEBSITE AND PROFESSIONAL ORGANIZATION

- American Organization of Nurse Executives (www.aone.org)

SIMULATION EDUCATIONAL SPECIALIST

264

BASIC DESCRIPTION

A nurse with a passion for education and simulation can become a simulation educational specialist. These nurses are responsible for identifying learning objectives and workforce goals and ensuring they are met through training sessions. They then work to plan, create, implement, and evaluate simulation-based learning with health care workers. Technological support and maintenance of simulation equipment may also be involved. They also can provide expert consultation and evaluation of these services. Employment can be found in hospitals or universities.

EDUCATIONAL REQUIREMENTS

RN preparation or other professional health care experience is required. A bachelor's degree in nursing or another health care–related field is necessary. A master's degree is preferred. Certification is encouraged and available through the Society for Simulation in Healthcare.

CORE COMPETENCIES/SKILLS NEEDED

- Experience with and understanding of simulation equipment
- Creative abilities to develop simulation-based scenarios
- Ability to educate through simulation training
- Ability to utilize technology and troubleshoot equipment
- Critical thinking and problem-solving skills
- Ability to remediate and effectively provide constructive feedback

RELATED WEBSITE AND PROFESSIONAL ORGANIZATION

- Society for Simulation in Healthcare (www.ssih.org)

265 SIMULATION LABORATORY DIRECTOR

BASIC DESCRIPTION
A simulation education director works in an academic setting and is responsible for managing daily simulation lab operations, designing and evaluating simulation cases based on educational principles, ensuring growth of the simulation program, updating programs or cases based on latest evidence, and conducting evaluation of the simulation program based on school and professional standard outcomes.

EDUCATIONAL REQUIREMENTS
A master's degree or higher is required; experience as a nurse educator is highly preferred.

CORE COMPETENCIES/SKILLS NEEDED
- Knowledge of budgeting, accounting, technology, and simulation software; equipment being used; quality improvement; regulations; and regulatory guidelines (patient safety guidelines)
- Excellent organizational, communication, leadership, and interpersonal skills
- Knowledge of adult-learning principles
- Strong clinical skills

RELATED WEBSITES AND PROFESSIONAL ORGANIZATIONS
- International Nursing Association for Clinical Simulation & Learning (www.inacsl.org/i4a/pages/index.cfm?pageid=1)
- National League for Nursing Simulation Innovation Resource Center (sirc.nln.org)
- Society for Simulation in Healthcare (www.ssih.org)

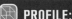

Simulation Center Director

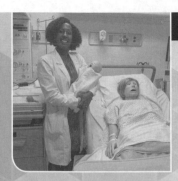

1. What is your educational background in nursing (and other areas) and what formal credentials do you hold?

I received my associate and bachelor's degrees in nursing. I continued my education and received a master's degree in nursing as a women's health nurse practitioner. Lastly, I obtained my Doctor of Nursing Practice with a focus on nursing education. I also have a certificate in simulation.

2. How did you first become interested in your current career?

My interest in simulation was sparked by a demonstration of SimMan and Birthing Noelle patient simulators at a conference. I have always been a person who loves technological gadgets and working with computers. About a year after I was introduced to simulation, a colleague recommended me for a part-time position at her institution as a simulation coordinator. The college received a grant to implement simulation, and I was hired to implement simulation into the nursing curriculum. After successfully implementing simulation into each medical–surgical course, I realized I was passionate about simulation education and wanted to purse a full-time position in the field of simulation education. Fortunately, I was able to find a full-time job as a director of simulation learning at a major university that utilizes simulation for 50% of its clinical hours. Our simulation center currently conducts over 100 simulation sessions a week for the undergraduate and graduate nursing programs.

3. What are the most rewarding aspects of your career?

My current position challenges me to develop new and innovative teaching strategies using simulation to enhance the education of our nursing students. In my role as director of one of the largest nursing simulation

Continued

programs in the country, the most rewarding aspect of my job is witnessing the effectiveness of simulation as an educational strategy. Simulation is the wave of the future in nursing education and I enjoy being in the forefront of the science of simulation learning. It is rewarding to hear from recent graduates that they value the positive impact simulation has played in their transition from nursing student to their role as an RN. Lastly, it is a pleasure offering my guidance and expertise in simulation education to other educators throughout the world.

4. What advice would you give to someone contemplating the same career path in nursing?

I would encourage everyone interested in simulation to expand their knowledge by attending conferences, reading journal articles, and training in the field of simulation. Joining organizations such as the International Nursing Association for Clinical Simulation and Learning and the Society for Simulation in Healthcare is an excellent way to network with other simulation experts and it provides a wealth of resources in the field of simulation. I would also encourage individuals to obtain training from experts in the field, such as those at Drexel University, or take advantage of recent graduate degree programs in simulation.

SPACE NURSE/ASTRONAUT

BASIC DESCRIPTION

Space nurses provide on-the-ground monitoring and a full range of health services to more than 400 astronauts, who are screened to determine if they meet the National Aeronautics and Space Administration (NASA) health requirements and, in some cases, military stipulations. These data must be meticulously documented because they are used to follow the health of astronauts throughout their lifetimes and to determine service eligibility, and are crucial to mission safety. Flight medicine clinic nurses also coordinate dietary and fitness services; clinic nurses staff a "sick call" service for astronauts to use before and after flight. At the first sign of physical discomfort, an astronaut first contacts a nurse, who administers appropriate treatment. Other nurses are employed as support staff for proctology and cardiovascular clinics and as instructors on the basis of self-assessment and medication administration for astronauts. Space Nurse Society members now meet at yearly conferences to exchange ideas, share research findings, and discuss the application of nursing methods used on Earth in space settings. Many members are nurse researchers who study the health risks associated with space travel.

EDUCATIONAL REQUIREMENTS

RN preparation is required; graduate preparation is required for researchers.

CORE COMPETENCIES/SKILLS NEEDED

- Excellent assessment skills
- Interest in, and knowledge of, aerospace industry and challenges
- Mental health skills
- Innovation and creativity
- Knowledge of physics and engineering

RELATED WEBSITES AND PROFESSIONAL ORGANIZATIONS

- Mars Society (www.marssociety.org)
- NASA (www.nasa.gov)

SPINAL CORD INJURY NURSE

BASIC DESCRIPTION

Spinal cord injury (SCI) nurses play a vital role in maintaining the patient's respiratory, gastrointestinal, urinary, musculoskeletal, and integumentary systems, and in providing psychological support to the patient and family. Caring for a patient with an SCI is complex and demanding. Although the primary focus in acute care management is directed toward sustaining life, it is critical that nurses involved in acute care management realize the effect their care has on the patient's rehabilitation and future life. By working to avoid preventable complications that cause additional morbidity and delay rehabilitation, nurses in acute care settings can help people with this devastating injury have the best possible opportunity to regain their health.

EDUCATIONAL REQUIREMENTS

RN preparation is required.

CORE COMPETENCIES/SKILLS NEEDED

- Excellent clinical skills
- Team skills for collaboration with respiratory and physical therapy to protect respiratory function
- Knowledge of the rehabilitation processes used in provision of care
- Good interpersonal skills
- Skills in helping patients and families manage anxiety by providing them with accurate information about the consequences of the injury in terms they can understand and by offering realistic hope for the future

RELATED WEBSITES AND PROFESSIONAL ORGANIZATIONS

- Academy of Spinal Cord Injury Professionals (www.academyscipro.org/Public/NursesMain.aspx)
- American Spinal Injury Association (asia-spinalinjury.org)

STAFF DEVELOPMENT EDUCATOR

BASIC DESCRIPTION

Staff development educators incorporate a variety of roles into the teaching of new staff members. They are responsible for the basic orientation and continuing education for new nurses and nursing staff employed by hospitals and other health care organizations. They monitor the overall staff compliance with clinical performance standards and participate in providing ongoing continuing education for nursing staff. They may specialize in certain clinical areas (e.g., gerontology, oncology) or they may be generalists. These educators function in a number of settings including hospitals, senior centers, clinics, health maintenance organizations, and schools of nursing.

EDUCATIONAL REQUIREMENTS

RN preparation is required; a Bachelor of Science or Master of Science in Nursing is preferred in some settings. Certification on Nursing Professional Development is available from the American Nurses Credentialing Center.

CORE COMPETENCIES/SKILLS NEEDED
- Ability to set priorities
- Knowledge of adult learning theory
- Ability to be an effective teacher
- Excellent communication skills
- Commitment to lifelong learning
- Ability to develop and implement lesson plans
- Staff development experience
- Positive attitude and enthusiasm for learning
- Ability to manage time effectively
- Ability to function autonomously

RELATED WEBSITES AND PROFESSIONAL ORGANIZATIONS
- American Nurses Credentialing Center (www.nursecredentialing.org)
- Association for Nursing Professional Development (www.anpd.org)

269 STAFF NURSE

BASIC DESCRIPTION
A staff nurse is a generalized job description of someone who works in a health care setting or facility. He or she works side by side with members of the health care team to treat and manage patients' conditions across age groups. Staff nurses' responsibilities are outlined by the employer.

EDUCATIONAL REQUIREMENTS
RN preparation is required; Bachelor of Science in Nursing is highly preferred.

CORE COMPETENCIES/SKILLS NEEDED
- Excellent communication and interpersonal skills
- Advanced knowledge based on area of specialization
- Knowledge of scope of nursing practice as defined by state board of nursing

RELATED WEBSITE AND PROFESSIONAL ORGANIZATION
- State Boards of Nursing

SUBACUTE-TRANSITION CARE NURSE

BASIC DESCRIPTION
Subacute or transition care nurses care for patients who have skilled care needs following an acute illness or hospitalization. Care could be rendered in a rehabilitation or skilled nursing facility or in a designated unit of a health care facility.

EDUCATIONAL REQUIREMENTS
RN preparation and basic life support certification are required.

CORE COMPETENCIES/SKILLS NEEDED
- Medical and surgical nursing experience
- Excellent assessment skills, and skill in the care of patients on intravenous therapy, ventilator, or tracheostomy
- Strong computer and documentation skills
- Ability to solve staffing difficulties when they arise
- Ability to work in a dynamic unit where patient admissions and discharges are high

RELATED WEBSITE AND PROFESSIONAL ORGANIZATION
- National Transitions of Care Coalition (ntocc.org/Home/tabid/55/Default.aspx)

271   SURGICAL NURSE PRACTITIONER

BASIC DESCRIPTION
A surgical nurse practitioner is an advanced practice nurse who works in a variety of surgical specialties with highly variable patient populations. The role of the surgical nurse practitioner goes from preparing the patient for surgical procedures by collecting a history and physical and interpreting diagnostic labs and imaging, to assisting surgeons during the surgical procedure, to managing pain and assisting with healing after the surgery, and to ensuring adequate follow-up care.

EDUCATIONAL REQUIREMENTS
RN preparation is required. A Master of Science in Nursing with advanced practice certification as a nurse practitioner is required. Certification is available through the American Association of Nurse Practitioners and the American Nurses Credentialing Center. Basic life support and advanced cardiac life support certifications are also necessary.

CORE COMPETENCIES/SKILLS NEEDED
- Extensive knowledge of surgical specialty in which the nurse practitioner is involved
- Risks and benefits of surgical procedures
- Training in surgical procedure specific to specialty
- Knowledge or appropriate preoperative and postoperative care

RELATED WEBSITES AND PROFESSIONAL ORGANIZATIONS
- Academy of Medical–Surgical Nurses (www.amsn.org)
- American Association of Nurse Practitioners (www.aanp.org)
- American Nurses Credentialing Center (www.nursecredentialing.org)
- American Society of periAnesthesia Nurses (www.aspan.org)
- Association of periOperative Registered Nurses (www.aorn.org)

BASIC DESCRIPTION

A talent acquisition leader works directly under the director for human resources to manage nurse recruiters to acquire new talent for an organization. He or she is responsible for developing recruitment strategies, developing relationships with talent sources, utilizing social media to advertise vacancies, analyzing turnover, and working with nursing management to meet employment qualifications.

EDUCATIONAL REQUIREMENTS

A bachelor's degree in nursing or health care–related field is required. A master's degree with clinical, leadership, and recruitment experience is highly preferred.

CORE COMPETENCIES/SKILLS NEEDED

- Ability to travel
- Ability to be highly organized
- Excellent communication skills
- Ability to network
- Strong interpersonal skills
- Ability to use social media
- Understanding of sourcing and recruitment strategies
- Leadership or managerial and health care experience

RELATED WEBSITES AND PROFESSIONAL ORGANIZATIONS

- National Association for Health Care Recruitment (www.nahcr.com)
- Nurse Recruiter for Nurses by Nurses (www.nurserecruiter.com)

273 TELEHEALTH NURSE

BASIC DESCRIPTION
Telehealth nurses conduct patient assessment, education, crisis intervention, counseling, and triage over the telephone or other forms of interactive media. They utilize care protocols, standards, and guidelines in arriving at decisions. They could be employed by home care agencies or insurance and medical groups.

EDUCATIONAL REQUIREMENTS
RN preparation is required; certification in telehealth nursing as part of ambulatory nursing is provided by the American Academy of Ambulatory Care Nursing.

CORE COMPETENCIES/SKILLS NEEDED
- Good communication skills
- Ability to sit for long periods
- Strong computer skills and ability to comfortably use computer-based guidelines
- Strong documentation skills using the electronic health/documentation record

RELATED WEBSITE AND PROFESSIONAL ORGANIZATION
- American Academy of Ambulatory Care Nursing (www.aaacn.org)

TELEMETRY NURSE 274

BASIC DESCRIPTION
Telemetry nurses assess acute changes in patients and work in a fast-paced environment. These nurses monitor the heart rhythm of patients in special care units of hospitals and analyze heart rhythms, interpret EKGs, note arrhythmias, and intervene in emergency situations.

EDUCATIONAL REQUIREMENTS
RN preparation is required. Certification as progressive care certified nurse is available from the American Association of Critical-Care Nurses Certification Corporation.

CORE COMPETENCIES/SKILLS NEEDED
- Excellent clinical skills
- Critical thinking ability
- Cardiovascular knowledge, including anatomy and physiology and cardiac disease processes
- Skill in teaching patients about medications, dietary changes, and postmyocardial infarction–activity restrictions
- Flexibility given the unpredictability of the patient's status
- Ability to use technology available for patient monitoring

RELATED WEBSITE AND PROFESSIONAL ORGANIZATION
- American Association of Critical-Care Nurses Certification Corporation (www.aacn.org)

275 TELEPHONE TRIAGE NURSE

BASIC DESCRIPTION
A telephone triage nurse provides a variety of services and information to patients over the phone. Most often, the telephone triage nurse uses written protocols to guide his or her practice, determine the urgency of care needed, and schedule appointments or direct callers to health care providers as needed. Accordingly, the goal of this unique form of nursing is to decrease unnecessary visits to physicians, nurse practitioners, and the emergency room as well as to provide information for self-care. Some triage nurses working for medical practices or clinics may be familiar with the patients and their health status. More often, though, the nurse must use his or her excellent communication and information-gathering skills to determine the best course of action for the patient. Triage nurses deal with the entire spectrum, from healthy patients to the acute and chronically ill. Triage nurses usually have regular hours but there is no direct patient contact, and triage nurses may spend long hours at a desk on the telephone and computer. There are opportunities to work in a variety of settings such as medical offices, health maintenance organizations, insurance companies, hospitals, clinics, and triage centers.

EDUCATIONAL REQUIREMENTS
RN preparation and a Bachelor of Science in Nursing are preferred. Previous emergency department or triage experience is highly desired for this role. Advanced cardiac life support and basic life support certifications are often required. Employers may require completion of Telehealth Nursing Practice Core Course.

CORE COMPETENCIES/SKILLS NEEDED
- Previous experience with triage, either on the telephone or in an emergency department
- Critical thinking skills
- Ability to determine the problem within the first few sentences of a conversation; a certain intuitive ability can be useful in assessing the situation and making the correct decision for the patient
- Superior verbal communication skills
- Strong assessment skills
- Excellent clinical skills
- Crisis intervention skills
- Typing and computer ability to keep track of information gathered during the telephone conversation

- Teaching ability, as patients may require instruction for self-care and/or symptom management
- Ability to remain calm in high-stress situations

RELATED WEBSITES AND PROFESSIONAL ORGANIZATIONS

- American Academy of Ambulatory Care Nursing (www.aaacn.org)
- Telephone Triage FAQs (teletriage.com/about-telephone-triage/faq-telephone-triage)

276 TRANSCULTURAL NURSE

BASIC DESCRIPTION
This advanced RN's role aims to expertly promote and provide culturally competent and congruent care to individuals, groups, and communities. This title also entails expertise in providing quality care based on transcultural nursing practices by transcultural nursing scholars.

EDUCATIONAL REQUIREMENTS
RN preparation is required. Educational preparation at the master's, postmaster's, or doctoral level is required for certification along with completion of one 3-credit course on cultural diversity or competence and 2,400 hours in transcultural nursing clinical practice, research, or teaching.

CORE COMPETENCIES/SKILLS NEEDED
- Ability to provide culturally sensitive and congruent care to diverse patient populations
- Knowledge of transcultural nursing theories and their applications
- Excellent communication skills
- Ability to work as part of a team

RELATED WEBSITES AND PROFESSIONAL ORGANIZATIONS
- American Association of Colleges of Nursing Cultural Competency (www.aacn.nche.edu/Education/cultural.htm)
- Transcultural Nursing Society (www.tcns.org)

TRANSPLANT NURSE

BASIC DESCRIPTION
The transplant nurse cares for recipient and living-donor patients throughout the transplantation process from end-stage disease processes to the preoperative, operative, and postoperative care. The transplant nurse is most often employed by the hospital with a transplant center. Practice roles can include nurse practitioner, case manager, transplant coordinator, research nurse, organ procurement nurse, and clinical specialist.

EDUCATIONAL REQUIREMENTS
RN preparation is required; a Bachelor or Master of Science in Nursing is often preferred.

CORE COMPETENCIES/SKILLS NEEDED
- Knowledge of transplant processes
- Excellent communication skills
- Teaching skills
- Knowledge of high-tech treatments
- Sensitivity in dealing with emotional and ethical issues
- Technological skills
- Ability to work with interdisciplinary teams

RELATED WEBSITES AND PROFESSIONAL ORGANIZATIONS
- International Society for Heart & Lung Transplantation (www.ishlt.org)
- International Transplant Nurses Society (www.itns.org)

278 TRANSPLANT NURSE PRACTITIONER

BASIC DESCRIPTION
Transplant nurse practitioners are advanced practice nurses who are experts in assessing, managing, and treating patients who require an organ transplant procedure or have received an organ transplant. They conduct history and physicals, order and interpret diagnostic tests, and manage preoperative and postoperative care management and coordination with an interdisciplinary team.

EDUCATIONAL REQUIREMENTS
RN preparation is required. A Master of Science in Nursing with advanced practice certification as a nurse practitioner is required. Certification is available through the American Association of Nurse Practitioners and the American Nurses Credentialing Center. Basic life support and advanced cardiac life support certifications are also necessary.

CORE COMPETENCIES/SKILLS NEEDED
- Extensive knowledge of transplant process, procedures, and postoperative management
- Ability to take a thorough history and physical and interpret diagnostic testing
- Expert knowledge in area of transplant
- Excellent teaching skills
- Sensitivity in dealing with emotional and ethical issues
- Ability to work as part of an interdisciplinary team

RELATED WEBSITES AND PROFESSIONAL ORGANIZATIONS
- American Association of Nurse Practitioners (www.aanp.org)
- American Nurses Credentialing Center (www.nursecredentialing.org)
- International Transplant Nurses Society (www.itns.org)
- Transplant Nurses' Association (www.tna.asn.au)

TRAUMA NURSE

BASIC DESCRIPTION

A trauma nurse cares for patients who have multisystem trauma across all age groups and works in acute care facilities and transport units.

EDUCATIONAL REQUIREMENTS

RN preparation and a Bachelor of Science in Nursing are preferred. Advanced cardiac life support, basic life support, pediatric advanced life support, and Trauma Course certifications are required; certification is offered by the Emergency Nurses Association.

CORE COMPETENCIES/SKILLS NEEDED

- Excellent clinical, critical thinking, and decision-making skills
- Knowledge of critical care and emergency medicine concepts across all age groups
- Ability to work in a dynamic high-stress environment
- Flexibility, motivation, and excellent communication and interpersonal skills
- Team player and excellent organizational skills

RELATED WEBSITE AND PROFESSIONAL ORGANIZATION

- Emergency Nurses Association (www.ena.org)

280 TRAVEL NURSE

BASIC DESCRIPTION

Travel nurses are those who take temporary nursing assignments, usually lasting 8 to 26 weeks (average is 13 weeks), in locations of the nurse's choice, in facilities across the United States and internationally. Travel nurses often work in hospital settings in staff nurse positions, but may also be found on cruise ships, in rural settings, or other roles that require the skill of an RN. A travel nurse works with an agency that makes arrangements for the position, provides accommodations at the location, and pays for travel expenses. The work activities depend on the location and the type of assignment. A nurse could go from a tertiary intensive care unit, caring for a postoperative coronary bypass patient, to a small 30-bed hospital where nurses care for a child with pneumonia next to an elderly patient with a stroke. Travel nurses are those who thrive on diversity and enjoy the opportunity to travel and experience new places and cultures.

EDUCATIONAL REQUIREMENTS

RN preparation is required; experience as a nurse is often preferred but not required.

CORE COMPETENCIES/SKILLS NEEDED

- Strong clinical skills; a critical care background is highly recommended, but not required
- Flexibility and adaptability
- Strong communication skills and the ability to get along with people to help integration within a unit and foster positive working relationships
- Adaptable to change

RELATED WEBSITES AND PROFESSIONAL ORGANIZATIONS

- NursesRx (www.nursesrx.com)
- Travel Nursing (www.travelnursing.org)
- Travel Nursing Blogs (travelnursingblogs.com)

...SE

BASIC DES...

A triage nur... ...rtment nurse who is responsible for conducting ... g a patient's clinical condition for the purpose of ... ...tient requires it. Although the triage nurse does ... , she may be required to deliver hands-on care if ...

EDUC...

RN pr... ...nce in Nursing are preferred. Previous emerg... ...ce is highly desired for this role; advanced cardi... certifications are required.

CO... ...NEEDED

...m-solving skills
...s situation that calls for quick thinking and

...ROFESSIONAL ORGANIZATIONS

...ritical-Care Nurses (www.aacn.org)
...ation (www.ena.org)

UNDERWRITER NURSE

BASIC DESCRIPTION

An underwriter nurse is responsible for assessing a patient's medical and insurance risks. Also, the underwriter nurse's medical and nursing backgrounds allow him or her to serve as a consultant to help insurance agents arrive at a patient's medical risk.

EDUCATIONAL REQUIREMENTS

RN preparation is required, and most positions require a Bachelor of Science in Nursing.

CORE COMPETENCIES/SKILLS NEEDED

- Good computer skills
- Excellent interpersonal and communication skills
- Excellent decision-making skills
- Thorough knowledge of health insurance industry

RELATED WEB SITE AND PROFESSIONAL ORGANIZATION

- Group Underwriters Association of America (www.guaa.com)

UNION DELEGATE/ REPRESENTATIVE

BASIC DESCRIPTION

A union is a group of employees who work together to make improvements in their workplace to achieve desired salaries, benefits, workplace safety, training, and resolution to other work-related issues. A nursing union delegate is an employee of a business institution who has a job and works among other employees of that institution. However, in addition to his or her day-to-day responsibilities, he or she has special training to represent the union within that hospital or organization. The union delegate's duties include resolving issues in the workplace; educating members regarding their rights, obligations, and benefits; representing members involved in disciplinary action; and organizing members to encourage involvement in the union events.

EDUCATIONAL REQUIREMENTS

RN preparation is required with relevant clinical experience with respect to unionized institution.

CORE COMPETENCIES/SKILLS NEEDED

- Strong communication and organizational skills
- Ability to advocate on behalf of union members
- Ability to defend rights of union members
- Well educated in respect to union contracts
- Ability to take initiative
- Excellent leadership skills

RELATED WEBSITES AND PROFESSIONAL ORGANIZATIONS

- Websites are available for various unions

284

UNION EXECUTIVE

BASIC DESCRIPTION
A union is a group of employees who work together to make improvements in their workplace to achieve desired salaries, benefits, workplace safety, training, and resolution to other work-related issues. In a nursing union, a union executive is a leader for the entire union, often at the state level. He or she works with union representatives from multiple hospitals or organizations to lead the union at the highest level. The union executive keeps union members updated with events and progress, organizes campaigns or rallies, and supports union members at the local level. Unlike a union delegate or union representative, the union executive does not work for an organization or hospital in which the union members are employed.

EDUCATIONAL REQUIREMENTS
RN preparation is required. A master's degree or leadership experience is preferred.

CORE COMPETENCIES/SKILLS NEEDED
- Excellent communication and organizational skills
- Knowledge of current best practices in nursing and politics
- Thorough understanding of respective union contracts
- Ability to take initiative
- Excellent leadership skills
- Creative and critical thinking skills

RELATED WEBSITES AND PROFESSIONAL ORGANIZATIONS
- Websites are available for various unions

BASIC DESCRIPTION

The university provost or president leads the faculty in fostering excellence in teaching and ensuring sound scholarship, clinical expertise, and research. The university president or provost articulates the vision of the university or school through leadership in school, university, and professional activities.

EDUCATIONAL REQUIREMENTS

PhD or EdD preparation is required.

CORE COMPETENCIES/SKILLS NEEDED

- Proven record of administrative leadership
- Experience in teaching nursing at a college or university level
- Grant-writing and/or research-funding skills and experience
- Scholarly publications to his or her credit
- Record of service to the community/profession commensurate with the rank of associate or full professor
- Excellent interpersonal skills
- Motivation (high energy)
- Ability to work with others
- Creativity
- Leadership

RELATED WEBSITES AND PROFESSIONAL ORGANIZATIONS

- American Nurses Credentialing Center (www.nursecredentialing.org)
- Sigma Theta Tau Honor Society of Nursing (www.nursingsociety.org)

286 UNIVERSITY VICE PRESIDENT (HEALTH SCIENCES)

BASIC DESCRIPTION
A university vice president works directly under the president or chancellor at an academic institution. This individual is responsible for several aspects of the university, including, but not limited to, overseeing large-scale finances, human resources, academic grounds and buildings, chairing academic or professional committees, surveillance of campus safety, involvement in academic affairs and research, management of information technology systems, serving as the chief administrative officer, overseeing and implementing strategic planning and programs, and supervising curriculum and schedule of the university. The university vice president also directly supervises the dean, faculty chairs, and other academic leaders in the institution.

EDUCATIONAL REQUIREMENTS
The minimum requirement for this position is a doctoral degree in nursing, business, or a health care–related field. Significant experience in educational administration is also required.

CORE COMPETENCIES/SKILLS NEEDED
- Excellent communication and interpersonal skills
- Ability to influence large numbers of people
- Proven record of administrative and/or academic leadership
- Scholarly publications to his or her credit
- Organizational skills and attention to detail
- Ability to negotiate contracts and agreements
- Strong leadership skills
- Ability to multitask and oversee multiple projects and activities
- Decisiveness
- Ability to collaborate
- Sound judgment and critical thinking skills
- Political sense
- Creativity
- Authority and attentiveness
- Financial skills and ability to budget

RELATED WEBSITES AND PROFESSIONAL ORGANIZATIONS
- American Association of Colleges of Nursing (www.aacn.nche.edu)
- National League for Nursing (www.nln.org)
- Sigma Theta Tau Society of Nursing (www.nursingsociety.org)

BASIC DESCRIPTION

Nurse practitioners who work in urgent care settings require an immense amount of knowledge and advanced skills. They care for patients of all ages with both acute and chronic health issues. They must be prepared to care for patients with minor injuries to major life-threatening events and be able to properly and safely manage them with appropriate referrals to the emergency department when necessary. They can order diagnostic tests to identify health problems and prescribe medications and treatments.

EDUCATIONAL REQUIREMENTS

RN preparation is required. A Master of Science in Nursing with advanced practice certification as a nurse practitioner is required. Certification is available through the American Association of Nurse Practitioners and the American Nurses Credentialing Center. Basic life support and advanced cardiac life support certifications are also necessary.

CORE COMPETENCIES/SKILLS NEEDED

- Expertise in emergency care
- Diagnostic testing interpretation skills
- Ability to perform minor procedures, such as suturing lacerations, draining of wounds, and splinting extremities
- EKG interpretation
- Ability to diagnose and manage acute health problems with appropriate referral to the emergency department when necessary
- Ability to function optimally in a fast-paced environment

RELATED WEBSITES AND PROFESSIONAL ORGANIZATIONS

- American Association of Nurse Practitioners (www.aanp.org)
- American Nurses Credentialing Center (www.nursecredentialing.org)
- Emergency Nurses Association (www.ena.org)

288 UROLOGY NURSE

BASIC DESCRIPTION
A urology nurse specializes in the care of patients who have urologic conditions, such as kidney stones, urinary tract infections, and cancers. They work in either inpatient or outpatient units. Aside from providing direct care, they also educate patients on preventing recurrences of acute conditions and avoiding complications.

EDUCATIONAL REQUIREMENTS
RN preparation and basic life support certification are required. A Bachelor of Science in Nursing is highly preferred; certification is offered by the Certification Board for Urologic Nurses and Associates.

CORE COMPETENCIES/SKILLS NEEDED
- Solid knowledge of the male and female urinary tract and reproductive systems, pathophysiology, and treatments
- Excellent bedside manner and sensitivity
- Strong computer and documentation skills

RELATED WEBSITES AND PROFESSIONAL ORGANIZATIONS
- American Urological Association (www.auanet.org)
- Certification Board for Urologic Nurses and Associates (www.cbuna.org)
- National Association for Continence (www.nafc.org)
- Society of Urologic Nurses and Associates (www.suna.org)

BASIC DESCRIPTION

Urology nurse practitioners are advanced practice nurses who specialize in urological health issues, such as prostate cancer, benign prostatic hyperplasia, or urinary incontinence. Their scope of work includes managing diseases, ordering and interpreting diagnostic imaging, and prescribing necessary medications for disease management. In some settings, they can also perform certain procedures, such as biopsies and cystoscopies. Urology nurse practitioners can work in inpatient or outpatient settings.

EDUCATIONAL REQUIREMENTS

RN preparation is required. A Master of Science in Nursing with advanced practice certification as a nurse practitioner is required. Certification is available through the American Association of Nurse Practitioners and the American Nurses Credentialing Center. Basic life support and advanced cardiac life support certifications are also necessary. Specialty certification in this field is available through the Certification Board for Urologic Nurses and Associates.

CORE COMPETENCIES/SKILLS NEEDED

- Ability to perform history and physical
- Expert knowledge of urologic diseases and treatment options
- Ability to collaborate with other specialties
- Ability to teach families and patients
- Excellent communication and interpersonal skills

RELATED WEBSITES AND PROFESSIONAL ORGANIZATIONS

- American Association of Nurse Practitioners (www.aanp.org)
- American Nurses Credentialing Center (www.nursecredentialing.org)
- American Urological Association (www.auanet.org)
- Certification Board for Urologic Nurses and Associates (www.cbuna.org)

290 UTILIZATION REVIEW NURSE

BASIC DESCRIPTION
A utilization review (UR) nurse examines and makes decisions about the appropriateness and level of patient care being provided. The eventual goal of UR nurses is to provide cost-effective care and ensure proper utilization of resources.

EDUCATIONAL REQUIREMENTS
RN preparation is required; a Bachelor of Science in Nursing is required in most positions. Certification in health care quality and management is offered by the American Board of Quality Assurance and Utilization Review Physicians.

CORE COMPETENCIES/SKILLS NEEDED
- Ability to work under stress and with autonomy
- Excellent organizational and leadership skills
- Excellent interpersonal and communication skills
- Experience in case management

RELATED WEBSITE AND PROFESSIONAL ORGANIZATION
- American Board of Quality Assurance and Utilization Review Physicians (www.abqaurp.org)

VACCINATION NURSE

BASIC DESCRIPTION
The vaccination or immunization nurse is responsible for providing vaccination to clients across age groups based on immunization guidelines and schedules, and federal, state, or county protocols.

EDUCATIONAL REQUIREMENTS
RN preparation is highly preferred in most states; basic life support certification is required.

CORE COMPETENCIES/SKILLS NEEDED
- Knowledge of vaccines–immunization schedule, correct anatomical sites, correct dosage, indications, contraindications, side effects, and steps to be taken during an anaphylactic reaction
- Knowledge of infection-control practices
- Excellent communication and customer-service orientation skills

RELATED WEBSITES AND PROFESSIONAL ORGANIZATIONS
- American Nurses Association (www.nursingworld.org)
- State Department of Health

292 VASCULAR NURSE

BASIC DESCRIPTION
The vascular nurse is responsible for nursing care of patients who have chronic vascular diseases, mostly seen in outpatient medical offices. A vascular nurse's job responsibility could include assisting the physician with treatment, minor surgical procedures, and administering medications.

EDUCATIONAL REQUIREMENTS
RN preparation is preferred; basic life support certification is required for most positions. Experience in a medical–surgical unit or critical care is highly desirable. Certification as cardiac vascular nurse is offered by the American Nurses Credentialing Center.

CORE COMPETENCIES/SKILLS NEEDED
- Astute assessment skills
- Excellent communication and interpersonal skills
- Good organizational and managerial skills as the job may include administrative responsibilities in the vascular clinic
- Computer literacy

RELATED WEBSITES AND PROFESSIONAL ORGANIZATIONS
- American Nurses Credentialing Center (www.nursecredentialing.org)
- Society for Vascular Nursing (www.svnnet.org)

VETERINARY NURSE

BASIC DESCRIPTION
A veterinary nurse works alongside a veterinarian in caring for animals. Job responsibilities vary from administering medications to treating wounds, performing tests, and conducting home pet visits. Areas of employment include animal laboratories, zoos, and organizations that protect the welfare of animals, such as the American Society for the Prevention of Cruelty to Animals.

EDUCATIONAL REQUIREMENTS
RN preparation is preferred.

CORE COMPETENCIES/SKILLS NEEDED
- Knowledge related to pet health
- Ability to work with members of the veterinary team
- Strong organizational skills as the job may also involve managerial responsibilities
- Strong intravenous skills

RELATED WEBSITE AND PROFESSIONAL ORGANIZATION
- American Society for the Prevention of Cruelty to Animals (www.aspca.org)

WELLNESS DIRECTOR

BASIC DESCRIPTION

A wellness director is responsible for managing health care needs and operations in a health care facility. He or she ensures that there is appropriate supervision of patients or residents and administrative duties are carried out, coordinates care, performs assessment of patient or facility needs, collaborates with support services, and trains staff. Employment is typically found in senior living centers or assisted living facilities.

EDUCATIONAL REQUIREMENTS

RN preparation is required. A Bachelor of Science in Nursing is required with relevant clinical experience.

CORE COMPETENCIES/SKILLS NEEDED

- Excellent communication skills
- Ability to pay attention to detail
- Compassion and attentiveness to needs of residents of facility
- Understanding of operations of a business
- Ability to be organized
- Ability to collaborate

RELATED WEBSITES AND PROFESSIONAL ORGANIZATIONS

There are no related websites or organizations.

BASIC DESCRIPTION
Wellness officers work with organizations to promote healthy lifestyles, offer education or life coaching, complete health screenings, define a wellness mission, and integrate wellness programs to benefit plans for the employees' gain. Wellness officers may work as part of management or in human resources in a variety of settings, such as academic facilities, business corporations, or hospitals.

EDUCATIONAL REQUIREMENTS
A bachelor's degree in a health-related field, such as nursing, is required. A graduate degree in nursing or health care–related field is preferred. Certification is available through numerous organizations and is highly recommended.

CORE COMPETENCIES/SKILLS NEEDED
- Knowledge of health-promotion and disease-prevention strategies
- Ability to screen for disease
- Coaching or experience in education
- Creativity
- Excellent communication and people skills
- Leadership or managerial skills
- Ability to be organized
- Ability to motivate

RELATED WEBSITES AND PROFESSIONAL ORGANIZATIONS
- National Association of Health Underwriters (www.nahu.org)
- National Commission for Health Education Credentialing, Inc. (www.nchec.org)
- National Wellness Institute (www.nationalwellness.org)
- Wellness Council of America (www.welcoa.org)

WOMEN'S HEALTH NURSE

BASIC DESCRIPTION

Women's health practitioners focus on primary care for women across the life span, from adolescence to the elderly. They may be prepared for basic nursing positions or as advanced practice nurses and provide services in hospitals and a range of primary care and community-based settings.

EDUCATIONAL REQUIREMENTS

RN preparation or advanced practice certification is required. Certification in various specialized women's health and primary care nursing is available from the National Certification Corporation for the Obstetric, Gynecological, and Neonatal Nursing Specialties.

CORE COMPETENCIES/SKILLS NEEDED

- Ability to perform well-woman assessments
- Knowledge to instruct on self-breast examinations and breast health education
- Knowledge of women's health
- Skill for patient education
- Ability to provide care to women across populations, social classes, and socio-economic and age groups, and in urban, suburban, and rural settings

RELATED WEBSITES AND PROFESSIONAL ORGANIZATIONS

- Association of Women's Health, Obstetric and Neonatal Nurses (www.awhonn.org)
- National Certification Corporation for the Obstetric, Gynecological, and Neonatal Nursing Specialties (www.nccwebsite.org)
- Nurse Practitioners in Women's Health (www.npwh.org)

BASIC DESCRIPTION

Working with women at different age groups, women's health nurse practitioners provide primary care for women who have gynecological, obstetrical, and family planning needs or issues. They also provide health education and counseling on issues that relate to women's health.

EDUCATIONAL REQUIREMENTS

RN preparation, nurse practitioner certification, and basic life support certification are required. Certification is offered by the National Certification Corporation.

CORE COMPETENCIES/SKILLS NEEDED

- Advanced knowledge that relates to obstetrical/gynecological assessment, pathophysiology, and its associated disease management
- Knowledge of unique needs of women
- Excellent communication and interpersonal skills
- Strong computer skills
- Strong organizational and leadership skills

RELATED WEBSITES AND PROFESSIONAL ORGANIZATIONS

- American Academy of Nurse Practitioners (www.aanp.org/AANPCMS2)
- National Certification Corporation (www.nccwebsite.org)
- Nurse Practitioners in Women's Health (www.npwh.org)

298 WOUND/OSTOMY/ CONTINENCE CARE NURSE PRACTITIONER

BASIC DESCRIPTION
The wound ostomy care nurse practitioner provides primary care to patients requiring ostomy and wound care that includes accurate assessment, documentation, treatment, and evaluation of care based on national standards and evidence-based guidelines. Aside from providing clinical services, the wound ostomy continence care nurse practitioner is also involved in patient teaching and care coordination to ensure timely recovery and discharge, and serving as a consultant to institutional and community partner organizations.

EDUCATIONAL REQUIREMENTS
RN preparation and nurse practitioner (NP) certification are required; most job positions require a 1-year experience as an NP and 5 years' experience as an RN; certification is available from the Wound Ostomy and Continence Nursing Certification Board.

CORE COMPETENCIES/SKILLS NEEDED
- Excellent assessment, interpersonal, and critical analysis skills
- Sensitivity to the needs of patients and their families
- Ability to work in a team
- Strong leadership and organizational skills
- Strong computer and documentation skills

RELATED WEBSITES AND PROFESSIONAL ORGANIZATIONS
- Wound Ostomy and Continence Nurses Society (www.wocn.org)
- Wound Ostomy and Continence Nursing Certification Board (www.wocncb.org/certification)

WOUND/OSTOMY/CONTINENCE NURSE

BASIC DESCRIPTION

A wound/ostomy/continence nurse is an RN specializing in the care of skin, particularly involving wounds, healing, and ostomy care and appliances. Hospitals and long-term care facilities employ most of the nurses, and some work in home care.

EDUCATIONAL REQUIREMENTS

RN preparation is required. Certification is available through the Wound Ostomy Continence Nursing Certification Board.

CORE COMPETENCIES/SKILLS NEEDED

- Excellent aseptic technique
- Excellent wound assessment skills and abilities, and wound care techniques
- Special knowledge of wound healing and skin physiology
- Ability to work independently and with a team
- Excellent documentation skills
- Knowledge of products, appliances, and wound healing
- Responsibility for dressing changes, assessment, selection of appropriate appliances, and topical wound healing, as well as pharmacological preparations
- Skill in teaching wound care and maintenance to other staff and patients
- Ability to maintain and promote ostomy care and teach patients to monitor their own appliances
- Skill in patient, family, and staff education
- Knowledge in maintaining photographic documentation

RELATED WEBSITES AND PROFESSIONAL ORGANIZATIONS

- Wound Ostomy and Continence Nurses Society (www.wocn.org)
- Wound Ostomy Continence Nursing Certification Board (www.wocncb.org)

300 WRITING/DOCUMENTATION COACH

BASIC DESCRIPTION
A nurse can function as a writing coach to work with clinical nurses to improve their documentation. A writing coach hosts workshops, directly mentors staff, and performs chart audits to help enhance quality of documentation. The coach can evaluate effectiveness pre- and postintervention to ensure documentation meets organizational, safety, and regulatory standards.

EDUCATIONAL REQUIREMENTS
RN preparation is required with relevant clinical experience. A graduate degree in nursing or related field is desired.

CORE COMPETENCIES/SKILLS NEEDED
- Coaching and teaching skills
- Excellent communication skills
- Attention to detail
- Ability to offer remediation and constructive criticism
- Advanced clinical knowledge
- Ability to work collaboratively

RELATED WEBSITES AND PROFESSIONAL ORGANIZATIONS
There are no related websites or organizations.

YOGA INSTRUCTOR/TRAINER 301

BASIC DESCRIPTION
A yoga instructor/trainer is a person who teaches the practice of yoga, which combines meditation, breath control, and various physical poses to promote wellness of the body and mind. Nurses who become yoga instructors can utilize their knowledge of health care to improve their practice and teach wellness to their students.

EDUCATIONAL REQUIREMENTS
Certification as a yoga instructor is required.

CORE COMPETENCIES/SKILLS NEEDED
- Excellent interpersonal and communication skills
- Excellent teaching and coaching skills
- Focus and attention to detail
- Dedication to yoga practice

RELATED WEBSITES AND PROFESSIONAL ORGANIZATIONS
- American Yoga Association (www.americanyogaassociation.org)
- International Association of Yoga Therapists (www.iayt.org)
- Yoga Alliance (www.yogaalliance.org)

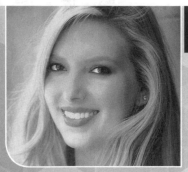

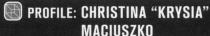

PROFILE: CHRISTINA "KRYSIA" MACIUSZKO

Yoga Instructor

1. What is your educational background in nursing (and other areas) and what formal credentials do you hold?

I received a Bachelor of Science in chemistry with a minor in biology and then completed a master's degree in nursing. I am currently working on my doctoral dissertation research for a PhD in integrative medicine.

2. How did you first become interested in your current career?

I started teaching group exercise classes while an undergraduate and continued to teach part time during graduate school. I started out teaching group step classes, then kickboxing, muscle conditioning, and Pilates. I received my yoga fitness certification in 2003, beginning my career as a yoga teacher. In 2005, I received my 200-Hour Yoga Teacher Training. This marked the start of my teaching outside of gyms, and in yoga studios. I taught yoga for the next 5 years, and in 2010 completed my 500-Hour Yoga Teacher Training. This achievement spurred my desire to open my own studio, and to teach teacher training at some point in the future. In 2011, I took a graduate course called "Advanced Leadership and Management in Nursing." We were assigned to write a business plan in the class. The faculty inspired and motivated me to open my yoga business sooner, rather than later. In late September 2012, I opened Krysia Energy Yoga, based on the business plan I had written in class. We offered our first yoga teacher training program almost immediately in January 2013. I designed a teaching program called Energy University 200-Hour Yoga Teacher Training, which includes nutrition, anatomy, yoga history, Ayurvedic medicine, sequencing, ethics, learning the Sanskrit language, and more. My goal is to offer a 500-hour Advanced Yoga Teacher Training Program at Energy University after I complete my PhD. This January, we are kicking off the brand-new signature training program that I designed, called Energy Core Barre. This is a unique class consisting of 30 minutes of traditional ballet barre exercises

Continued

PROFILE: CHRISTINA "KRYSIA" MACIUSZKO
Continued

followed by 30 minutes of Pilates exercises on the mat, ending with yoga stretching. It is an incredible experience of authentic grace, fun sequencing, and great toning exercises.

3. What are the most rewarding aspects of your career?

Recently, I had an exciting opportunity to teach yoga at a resort in Mexico. The teacher training program I designed was approved by Yoga Alliance, the international certifying body for yoga teachers and yoga teacher training. This seal of approval can literally open doors for a yoga teacher or trainer all over the world. I plan to return to Mexico to teach again next year, and I would still love to experience yoga or yoga training in India someday. In the meantime, I am grateful that I love what I do, and that I own my own business. I refuse to call it work. If people ask me when I'm "working", I always change the verbiage to, "Do you mean when am I teaching?" If I view it as work then I might want to quit someday, so I don't view it as work. I love what I do, and I look forward to seeing my students every day. I plan for Krysia Energy Yoga to thrive, and to be successful, for many years to come. I will continue to do my best to keep Krysia Energy Yoga innovative and as forward thinking as possible. This year, in 2016, we proudly released our very own Krysia Energy Yoga mobile application, available in the app store for iPhone or in the Google Play store for Android devices.

4. What advice would you give to someone contemplating the same career path in nursing?

The knowledge I have gained through nursing school has been extremely valuable and helpful to me. Nursing education can be practical, as well as philosophical, just like yoga is. Nursing teaches caring and compassion, as well as how to make positive changes, or experience a transformation. I use these foundational elements of nursing on a daily basis as a yoga teacher and a healer. I would advise someone contemplating a career path in nursing to consider thinking outside the box. Be creative, "think different" as Steve Jobs would say. Think big, and remember, the possibilities are endless, and limitless, not finite or limited. As Joseph Campbell once said, "Follow your bliss and doors will open." Be confident, prepared, as well as willing to take certain calculated risks in order to progress forward and to stay relevant.

SPECIALTY CERTIFICATION BOARD AND CONTACT INFORMATION

ACADEMIC NURSE EDUCATOR
National League for Nursing
www.nln.org/FacultyCertification/index.htm

ACUTE CARE NURSE PRACTITIONER
American Nurses Credentialing Center
www.nursecredentialing.org

ADDICTIONS NURSING
International Nurses Society on Addictions
intnsa@intnsa.org; www.intnsa.org

ADULT NURSES
Adult Health Clinical Nurse Specialist
American Nurses Credentialing Center
www.nursecredentialing.org

Adult Nurse Practitioner
American Nurses Credentialing Center
www.nursecredentialing.org

Adult Psychiatric and Mental Health
Clinical Nurse Specialist
American Nurses Credentialing Center
www.nursecredentialing.org

Adult Psychiatric and Mental Health Nurse Practitioner
American Nurses Credentialing Center
www.nursecredentialing.org

AMBULATORY CARE NURSING
American Nurses Credentialing Center
www.nursecredentialing.org

CARDIOVASCULAR NURSING
American Nurses Credentialing Center
www.nursecredentialing.org

CASE MANAGEMENT NURSING
American Nurses Credentialing Center
www.nursecredentialing.org

CRITICAL CARE NURSING
American Association of Critical-Care
www.certcorp.org

Adult Critical-Care Nurse
AACN Certification Corporation
www.certcorp.org

Cardiac Medicine Certification
AACN Certification Corporation
www.certcorp.org

Clinical Nurse Specialist in Acute and Critical Care; Adult, Neonatal, or Pediatric
AACN Certification Corporation
www.certcorp.org

Neonatal Critical-Care Nurse
AACN Certification Corporation
www.certcorp.org

Pediatric Critical-Care Nurse
AACN Certification Corporation
www.certcorp.org

Progressive Care Certified Nurse
AACN Certification Corporation
www.certcorp.org

DIABETES EDUCATORS
National Certification Board for Diabetes Educators
www.ncbde.org

EMERGENCY NURSING
Board of Certification for Emergency Nursing
www.ena.org/bcen

FAMILY NURSES
Family Nurse Practitioner
American Nurses Credentialing Center
www.nursecredentialing.org

Appendix: Specialty Certification Board and Contact Information

Family Psychiatric and Mental Health Nurse Practitioner
www.nursecredentialing.org

FLIGHT NURSING
Board of Certification for Emergency Nursing
www.ena.org/bcen

GASTROENTEROLOGY
American Board of Certification for Gastroenterology
www.abcgn.org

GENETICS NURSING
Advanced Practice Nurse in Genetics
www.geneticnurse.org

Genetics Clinical Nurse
Advanced Practice Nurse in Genetics
Genetic Nursing Credentialing Commission, Inc.
www.geneticnurse.org

GERONTOLOGY NURSES
Gerontological Nursing
American Nurses Credentialing Center
www.nursecredentialing.org

Gerontological Nurse Practitioner
American Nurses Credentialing Center
www.nursecredentialing.org

Gerontology Clinical Nurse Specialist
American Nurses Credentialing Center
www.nursecredentialing.org

HEALTHCARE QUALITY
Applied Measurement Professionals
www.cphq.org

HIV/AIDS NURSING
AIDS Certified Registered Nurse
HIV/AIDS Nursing Certification Board
www.hancb.org

HOLISTIC NURSING
American Holistic Nurses' Certification Corp.
www.ahncc.org

HOSPICE AND PALLIATIVE NURSING
Advanced Certified Hospice and Palliative Nurse
www.nbchpn.org

Certified Hospice and Palliative Care Administrator
National Board for Certification of Hospice and Palliative Nurses
www.nbchpn.org

Certified Hospice and Palliative Nurse
National Board for Certification of Hospice and Palliative Nurses
www.nbchpn.org

Certified Hospice and Palliative Licensed Nurse
National Board for Certification of Hospice and Palliative Nurses
www.nbchpn.org

Certified Hospice and Palliative Nursing
National Board for Certification of Hospice and Palliative Nurses
www.nbchpn.org

INFECTION CONTROL
Certification Board of Infection Control and Epidemiology, Inc.
www.cbic.org

INFORMATICS
American Nurses Credentialing Center
www.nursecredentialing.org

INFUSION NURSING
Infusion Nurses Certification Corporation
www.incc1.org

LACTATION CONSULTANT
International Board of Lactation Consultant Examiners
www.iblce.org

LEGAL NURSE CONSULTING
American Legal Nurse Consultant Certification Board
www.aalnc.org

MANAGED CARE NURSING
American Board of Managed Care Nursing
www.abmcn.org

MEDICAL-SURGICAL NURSING
American Nurses Credentialing Center
www.nursecredentialing.org

Academy of Medical Surgical Nurses
www.medsurgnurse.org

MS Nurses International Certification Board
www.ptcny.com

NEPHROLOGY NURSING
Board of Nephrology Examiners Nursing and
Technology (BONENT)
www.bonent.org

Nephrology Nursing Certification Commission
www.nncc-exam.org

NEUROSCIENCE NURSING
American Board of Neuroscience Nursing
www.aann.org

**NURSE ADMINISTRATION—LONG-TERM
CARE (LTC)**
NADONA/LTC Certification Registrar
www.nadona.org

NURSE ANESTHETIST
National Board on Certification and Recertification of
Nurse Anesthetists
www.nbcrna.org

NURSE EXECUTIVE
American Nurses Credentialing Center
www.nursecredentialing.org

NURSE EXECUTIVE, ADVANCED
American Nurses Credentialing Center
www.nursecredentialing.org

NURSE MIDWIFERY AND MIDWIFERY
American Midwifery Certification Board
www.amcbmidwife.org

NURSES IN NUTRITION SUPPORT
National Board of Nutrition Support Certification
www.nutritioncertify.org

NURSING PROFESSIONAL DEVELOPMENT
American Nurses Credentialing Center
www.nursecredentialing.org

OCCUPATIONAL HEALTH NURSING
Occupational Health Nurse Case Manager
American Board for Occupational Health Nurses, Inc.
www.abohn.org

Occupational Health Safety Manager
American Board for Occupational Health Nurses, Inc.
www.abohn.org

ONCOLOGY NURSING
Oncology Nursing Certification Corporation
www.oncc.org

OPHTHALMIC NURSING
National Certifying Board for Ophthalmic Registered
Nurses
www.asorn.org

ORTHOPAEDIC NURSING
www.oncb.org

**OTORHINOLARYNGOLOGY AND HEAD-NECK
NURSES**
www.sohnnurse.com

PAIN MANAGEMENT
American Nurses Credentialing Center
www.nursecredentialing.org

American Academy of Pain Management
www.aapainmanage.org

PEDIATRIC NURSES
American Nurses Credentialing Center
www.nursecredentialing.org

Pediatric Nursing Certification Board (PNCB)
www.pncb.org

Pediatric Nurse Practitioner
American Nurses Credentialing Center
www.nursecredentialing.org

PEDIATRIC ONCOLOGY
Oncology Nursing Certification Corporation
www.oncc.org

Appendix: Specialty Certification Board and Contact Information

PERIANESTHESIA NURSING
American Board of PeriAnesthesia Nursing
Certification, Inc.
www.cpancapa.org

PERIOPERATIVE NURSING
Competency and Credentialing Institute
www.cc-institute.org

RN First Assistant
Competency and Credentialing Institute
www.cc-institute.org

PLASTIC AND RECONSTRUCTIVE SURGICAL NURSING
American Society of Plastic Surgery Nurses
www.aspsn.org

PSYCHIATRIC AND MENTAL HEALTH NURSING
American Nurses Credentialing Center
www.nursecredentialing.org

ADVANCED PUBLIC HEALTH NURSE
American Nurses Credentialing Center
www.nursecredentialing.org

RADIOLOGIC NURSING
Radiologic Nursing Certification Board, Inc.
www.arinursing.org

REHABILITATION NURSING
Rehabilitation Nursing Certification Board
www.rehabnurse.org

SCHOOL NURSING
National Board for Certification of School Nurses
www.nbcsn.com

SEXUAL ASSAULT NURSE EXAMINER—ADULT/ ADOLESCENT
Forensic Nursing Certification Board
www.iafn.org

UROLOGY NURSING
Certification Board for Urologic Nurses and Associates
(CBUNA)
www.suna.org

WOMEN'S HEALTH/PRIMARY CARE NURSING
Electronic Fetal Monitoring
Inpatient Obstetric Nurse
Low-Risk Neonatal Nurse
Maternal Newborn Nurse
Neonatal Intensive Care Nurse
Neonatal Nurse Practitioner
Women's Healthcare Nurse
National Certification Corporation for the Obstetric,
Gynecological, and Neonatal
Specialties National Certification Corporation
www.nccwebsite.org

WOUND, OSTOMY, AND CONTINENCE NURSING
Wound, Ostomy, and Continence Nursing Certification
Board
www.wocncb.org

Source: Adapted from "Your Guide to Certification," *American Journal of Nursing*, January 1, 2012, Vol. 42, Issue 1, pp. 43–55. New York, NY: Wolters Kluwer Health.

GLOSSARY OF ACRONYMS

AANP	American Association of Nurse Practitioners
AAPC	American Association of Professional Coders
ABGC	American Board of Genetic Counseling
ACLS	advanced cardiac life support
AD	associate degree
ANA	American Nurses Association
ANCC	American Nurses Credentialing Center
AORN	Association of periOperative Registered Nurses
APRN	advanced practice registered nurse
BLS	basic life support
BMT	bone marrow transplant
BSN	Bachelor of Science in Nursing
CARN	certified addictions registered nurse
CCRN	critical care registered nurse
CDC	Centers for Disease Control and Prevention
CEO	chief executive officer
CHPN	Certified Hospice and Palliative Care Nurse
CIA	Central Intelligence Agency
CMS	Centers for Medicare & Medicaid Services
CNRN	Certified Neuroscience Registered Nurse
CNS	clinical nurse specialist
COO	chief operating officer
CPHQ	certified professional in health care quality
CPR	cardiopulmonary resuscitation
CPT	Current Procedural Terminology
CRNA	certified registered nurse anesthetist
CRRN	certified rehabilitation registered nurse
DNP	Doctorate of Nursing Practice
ED	emergency department
EMT	emergency medical technician
ENT	ear, nose, and throat
ER	emergency room
FDA	Food and Drug Administration
FNP	family nurse practitioner
ICD	International Classification of Diseases
ICU	intensive care unit

IUI	intrauterine insemination
IVF	in vitro fertilization
JD	juris doctor
LNC	legal nurse consultant
MDS	minimum data set
MPH	Master's in Public Health
MSN	Master of Science in Nursing
NALS	neonatal advanced life support
NICU	neonatal intensive care unit
NNP	neonatal nurse practitioner
NP	nurse practitioner
ONCC	Oncology Nursing Certification Corporation
OSHA	Occupational Safety and Health Administration
PALS	pediatric advanced life support
PRI	patient review instrument
PTAP	Practice Transition Accreditation Program
RDN	registered diet nutritionist
RD	registered dietician
RNFA	registered nurse first assist
RN	registered nurse
SANE	sexual assault nurse examiner
SNF	skilled nursing facilities
TB	tuberculosis
TJC	The Joint Commission
UAP	unlicensed assistive personnel
UR	utilization review

INDEX